Advances in Tracheal Intubation

Edited by Jessica A. Lovich-Sapola, Kelly Lebak, Michael D. Bassett and Kasia P. Rubin

Published in London, United Kingdom

Advances in Tracheal Intubation
http://dx.doi.org/10.5772/intechopen.102176
Edited by Jessica A. Lovich-Sapola, Kelly Lebak, Michael D. Bassett and Kasia P. Rubin

Contributors
Hsiang-Ning Luk, Jason Zhensheng Qu, Alan Henry Shikani, Hsuan-Nu Luk, Glenardi Glenardi, Ajay Singh, Rekha Gupta, Naveen B Naik, Shiv Lal Soni, Venkata Ganesh, Kashish Garg, Ankita Dhir, Narender Kaloria, Jessica A. Lovich-Sapola, Kasia P. Rubin, William Pender, Kelly Lebak

First published in London, United Kingdom, 2023 by IntechOpen
IntechOpen is the global imprint of INTECHOPEN LIMITED, registered in England and Wales, registration number: 11086078, 5 Princes Gate Court, London, SW7 2QJ, United Kingdom

British Library Cataloguing-in-Publication Data
A catalogue record for this book is available from the British Library

Additional hard and PDF copies can be obtained from orders@intechopen.com

Advances in Tracheal Intubation
Edited by Jessica A. Lovich-Sapola, Kelly Lebak, Michael D. Bassett and Kasia P. Rubin
p. cm.
Print ISBN 978-1-80356-860-7
Online ISBN 978-1-80356-861-4
eBook (PDF) ISBN 978-1-80356-862-1

Meet the editors

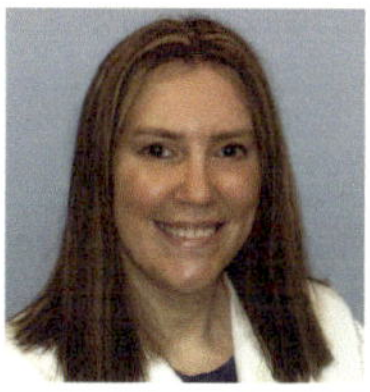

Jessica Lovich-Sapola is a professor at the Cleveland Clinic Lerner College of Medicine, a division of Case Western Reserve University School of Medicine, USA. She is also a board-certified anesthesiologist at the Cleveland Clinic. She obtained her MD from Northeast Ohio Medical University, USA, and MBA from Cleveland State University, USA. She is a fellow of the American Society of Anesthesiologists (ASA). Her academic focus is on trauma, burn, and regional anesthesia. She has authored 5 peer-reviewed articles, more than 100 book chapters, and more than 20 abstracts presented at national meetings. She is also the editor of the first and second editions of *Anesthesia Oral Board Review: Knocking Out the Boards*. She serves on committees for the Ohio Society of Anesthesiologists (OSA) and the Society for Ambulatory Anesthesia (SAMBA).

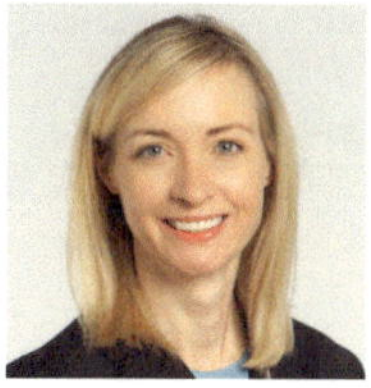

Kasia Rubin is a board-certified anesthesiologist at Cleveland Clinic Foundation skilled in regional anesthesia, quality management, medical writing, and pediatrics. She completed her MD at Case Western Reserve University School of Medicine, USA, in 2013 and an MBA at Indiana University, Kelley School of Business, USA, in 2017. She completed her anesthesiology fellowship at the MetroHealth Medical Center, USA, and a pediatric anesthesiology fellowship at Cincinnati Children's Hospital Medical Center, USA. She is Assistant Professor of Anesthesiology at Cleveland Clinic Lerner College of Medicine, USA, as well as an active member of the American Board of Anesthesiology and Society of Pediatric Anesthesia.

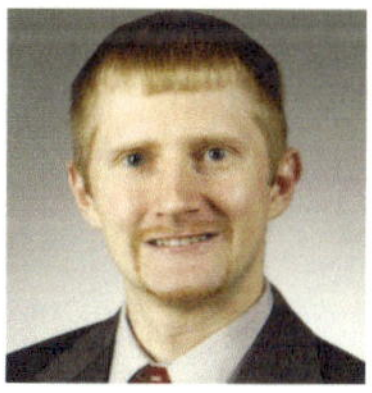

Michael Bassett is an Assistant Professor of Anesthesiology at Case Western Reserve University School of Medicine, USA. He completed his medical doctorate at the University of Toledo College of Medicine, USA, and his bachelor of science at The Ohio State University, USA. He is currently a board-certified anesthesiologist at MetroHealth Medical Center, USA, with expertise in trauma and regional anesthesia. He is the assistant program director of the residency program and is in charge of the medical student electives. He has authored several book chapters and is a committee member of the Ohio Society of Anesthesiology.

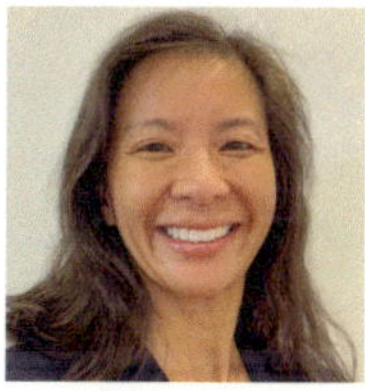

Kelly Lebak is a board-certified anesthesiologist at MetroHealth Medical Center, USA, and is an assistant professor at Case Western Reserve University School of Medicine, USA. She completed an ambulatory anesthesiology fellowship at the University of Wisconsin-Madison, USA. She is the medical director for MetroHealth's three ambulatory surgery centers and is active on residency committees. She is an active member of the American Society of Anesthesiologists and on multiple committees in the Ohio Society of Anesthesiologists and Society for Ambulatory Anesthesia.

Contents

Preface

Tracheal intubation is one of the cornerstones of anesthesiology. To the layperson, and even many surgeons, intubation appears to be a somewhat simple procedure. Indeed, intubation is easy 95% of the time. The incidence of difficult direct laryngoscopy these days is about 5%, with rates of difficult or failed intubation much lower.

This book is a reference tool that presents the most up-to-date information on advances in tracheal intubation. Chapters discuss advanced tracheal intubation techniques such as video laryngoscopy, ultrasound use for airway management, the video-assisted intubating stylet technique, and airway management techniques for obstetric patients. All the chapters highlight the advances, successes, and continued challenges that we face with tracheal intubation. It is our hope that the information contained herein will help practitioners achieve 100% success with endotracheal tube placement.

Jessica A. Lovich-Sapola, MD, MBA, FASA
and Kasia P. Rubin, MD, MBA, FASA
Cleveland Clinic,
Cleveland, Ohio, USA

Michael D. Bassett, MD and Kelly Lebak, MD, FASA
MetroHealth Medical Center,
Cleveland, Ohio, USA

Chapter 1

Introductory Chapter: Advances in Tracheal Intubation

Kelly Lebak

1. Introduction

Tracheal intubation is one of the cornerstones of anesthesiology. To the lay person, and even our surgical colleagues, it should not be that difficult ...just put a narrow tube in the trachea; no big deal. Indeed, we as a profession make it look easy, and 95% of the time it is. The incidence of difficult direct laryngoscopy these days is only 4.9% [1] with difficult or failed intubation much lower than this at 0.33% and 0.01% respectively [2]. This book will look at four different aspects of advanced tracheal intubation including videolaryngoscopy, ultrasound use for airway management, the video-assisted intubating stylet technique, and airway management in obstetrics.

Without question, videolaryngoscopy (VL) has changed the practice of endotracheal tube (ETT) placement and the practice of anesthesiology. Much of the time, VL makes ETT placement look easy (to the lay person). First introduced in 2001 [3], it has grown ubiquitous in ETT placement. In fact, aside from "practice" or the need to "keep our skills up," do many/any of us, who grew up in the days of direct laryngoscopy (DL) or early days of VL, DL anymore? Can anyone imagine how we intubated patients with "anterior" cords atraumatically? Given all the advantages of VL including successful ETT placement in difficult airways, multiple clinicians' ability to view the airway, and documentation of airway findings, it is no wonder that VL has gained a prominent place in the American Society of Anesthesiologists Practice Guidelines of Difficult Airway Management [4]. There are still disadvantages with VL, namely the dreaded "blind zone" where injuries can occur, a bulkier design if a channeled blade is used, and increased cost compared with DL, but it has forever changed the practice of ETT placement.

VL is one of the indispensable tools in our arsenal, and ultrasound may be the next. It is commonly used by anesthesiologists for invasive line placements, nerve blocks, and point-of-care ultrasound. Not surprisingly, given its success in these realms, it is starting to be used for airway management. There is work being done using the US to predict difficult mask ventilation or intubation by measuring tongue thickness or soft tissue thickness at the vocal cords, predict proper ETT size in pediatric patients or patients with obesity, identification of airway nerves for awake fiberoptic blocks, identification of upper airway inflammation including epiglottitis and sinusitis (useful for nasal ETT placement), guidance of the ETT to the correct depth in the trachea, confirmation of ETT and supraglottic airway placement, lung ultrasound as an indirect sign of correct ETT placement, surgical airway guidance via visualization of the cricothyroid membrane and trachea, and evaluation of other pulmonary pathology including pneumothorax.

IntechOpen

When faced with a difficult airway, anesthesiologists have multiple tools from which to choose. A lesser-known tool is a video-assisted intubating stylet (VS) which is simple, portable, and easy to use. It can be used for the Shikani technique for intubation. The Shikani optical stylet is a bendable stylet with an endoscope at the distal tip that is used to visually guide the ETT. The Shikani method of intubation uses this stylet for guidance while grasping the mandible to lift the jaw anteriorly and advances the ETT and stylet combination into the larynx with direct visualization from the stylet. This technique negates: the need for a laryngoscope, increased forces on dentition, or cervical spine extension. An endoscopic stylet was first introduced in 1979 and now multiple similar video-assisted stylets are on the market. They can be used for various ETTs including regular ETTS, laser, and double-lumen tubes. Advantages of using VS include both the ease of obtaining a superior glottic view and placing the ETT through the viewed glottis. Potential drawbacks are lens fogging and secretions obscuring the view (though not exclusive to VS). It can be combined with DL and VL which is particularly useful in difficult airways as it uses the strengths of both modalities in that DL/VL is used to open the airway and lift the epiglottis allowing the VS to sneak under the epiglottis and obtain an optimized glottic view. Due to its many advantages, VS can not only be in the anesthesiologist's arsenal of difficult airway tools, but also for every day and every airway use in both adults and pediatric patients.

Despite the many advances to manage airways that our specialty has seen over the last several decades, airways in pregnancy (particularly in parturients) still elude us. Indeed, the incidence of failed intubation in pregnancy has not changed in 40 years. Airway complications are the leading causes of anesthesia-related maternal mortality with an incidence of failed intubation at 1 in 390 [5]. Multiple physiologic and anatomical changes put obstetric patients at risk for airway complications including airway changes due to edema particularly during labor and delivery, reduced functional residual capacity to closing capacity and increased oxygen demand resulting in faster onset of hypoxemia at induction, increased gastric pressure and relative incompetence of the lower esophageal sphincter, prolonged gastric emptying time during labor, pregnancy-related weight gain, and breast enlargement.

We must mitigate those changes with what we have until technology can be developed to magically (or at least competently) intubate during pregnancy 100% of the time. At this time in our arsenal, we can: do a preanesthetic airway assessment (sometimes under the duress of time), have an induction plan and multiple backup plans, be familiar with algorithms for difficult airways in pregnancy, premedicate to reduce pH and reduce gastric volume, perform rapid sequence inductions or positive pressure ventilation with cricoid pressure likely with VL and a relatively smaller, cuffed endotracheal tube with an introducer, and lastly, consider a second generation supraglottic airway and proceed with surgery if unable to intubate. In the case of "can't intubate, can't oxygenate," laryngospasm should be quickly ruled out, and then proceed with either a tracheotomy or cricothyrotomy.

All four of the following chapters highlight the advances, successes, and continued challenges that we face with tracheal intubation. The hope that we have with this book is that with widespread education and new technology eventually we can make ETT placement look easy 100% of the time.

Author details

Kelly Lebak
MetroHealth Medical Center, Cleveland, Ohio, USA

*Address all correspondence to: kellylebak@gmail.com

References

[1] Heinrich S, Birkholz T, Irouschek A, Ackermann A, Schmidt J. Incidences and predictors of difficult laryngoscopy in adult patients undergoing general anesthesia: A single-center analysis of 102,305 cases. Journal of Anesthesia. 2013;**27**(6):815-821. DOI: 10.1007/s00540-013-1650-4 Epub 2013 Jun 9

[2] Schroeder RA, Pollard R, Dhakal I, Cooter M, Aronson S, Grichnik K, et al. Temporal trends in difficult and failed tracheal intubation in a regional community anesthetic practice. Anesthesiology. 2018;**128**:502-510. DOI: 10.1097/ALN.0000000000001974

[3] https://das.uk.com/content/2015-das-medal-john-a-pacey

[4] Apfelbaum JL, Hagberg CA, Connis RT, Abdelmalak BB, Agarkar M, Dutton RP, et al. 2022 American Society of Anesthesiologists Practice Guidelines for Management of the Difficult Airway. Anesthesiology. 2022;**136**:31-81. DOI: 10.1097/ALN.0000000000004002

[5] Kinsella SM, Winton AL, Mushambi MC, Ramaswamy K, Swales H, Quinn AC, et al. Failed tracheal intubation during obstetric general anaesthesia: A literature review. International Journal of Obstetric Anesthesia. 2015;**24**(4):356-374

Chapter 2

Video-Assisted Laryngoscopy and Its Effects on Difficult Airway Management

William Pender, Jessica A. Lovich-Sapola and Kasia P. Rubin

Abstract

Video-assisted laryngoscopy (VL) has become a critical tool in the anesthesiologist's arsenal. Compared with direct laryngoscopy (DL), VL often improves laryngeal views, increases the frequency of first-attempt intubations, and decreases the time in achieving successful intubation. First-line utilization of VL has changed the approach to airway management, with some specialists indicating that VL will eventually replace traditional DL. In this chapter, we describe the history of video laryngoscopy, the advantages and disadvantages of currently available VL technologies, and its emerging utility in a variety of clinical settings.

Keywords: laryngoscopy, video laryngoscopy, tracheal intubation, airway management, airway management techniques

1. Introduction

The techniques for managing a patient's airway are constantly evolving. Historically, direct visualization of the vocal cords and related airway structures was required for each laryngoscopy. However, advances in technology have allowed for indirect laryngoscopy. Simply put, this technique involves visualizing the patient's vocal cords without utilizing a direct line of site. Various forms of indirect laryngoscopy exist including fiberoptic bronchoscopes, fiberoptic stylets, mirror or prism optically enhanced laryngoscopes, and video laryngoscopes – the focus of this chapter. By using a laryngoscope equipped with a light source and video camera, a provider can visualize structures not within direct line of sight. The GlideScope®, developed in 1999 with the support of Dr. Jack Pacey, was the first video laryngoscope to be readily available. Since then, many different video laryngoscopes have been developed, each with its own advantages and disadvantages. In this chapter, we discuss the advantages and disadvantages of video laryngoscopy, differences in technique compared to direct laryngoscopy (DL), risks and benefits, various devices available, and what the current literature tells us about this airway technique compared to other utilized techniques.

2. Types of video laryngoscopes

As previously stated, the GlideScope® was the first readily available video laryngoscope. Today, many variations of video laryngoscopes exist, each with its own advantages and disadvantages when compared to one another. Video laryngoscopes can be broken down by two categories: blade type and whether they are channeled. Two main types of blades exist: the Macintosh blade and the acute-angle blade. Macintosh blades maintain the traditional shape as used in direct laryngoscopy. Acute-angle blades, as the name suggests, are hyper-angulated to allow for better anterior visualization. Channeled scopes are shaped to match the anatomic curve of the upper airway and the built-in channel provides a guided passage for the endotracheal tube. The different blade types and presence of a channel offer different advantages and disadvantages.

Examples of available Macintosh-style blades include the GlideScope®, Storz C-MAC (single and reusable), and McGRATH™ (single use). An advantage of these blades is most providers are familiar with this style of blade in terms of its shape and technique for use. The blade is shaped with the same angle as a direct laryngoscope. The provider follows the same initial steps for airway management including patient positioning, mouth opening, rightward insertion of blade, sweeping of the tongue, and direct advancement past the soft palate. At this point, the provider can continue use of this blade for direct visualization or indirectly visualize the airway using the device-specific video source. The blade is either directly or indirectly guided into the vallecula, and the epiglottis is lifted to expose the vocal cords. The provider directly visualizes the endotracheal tube entering the mouth and advancement past the soft palate after which the provider again has the choice of either directly or indirectly viewing the advancement of the tube through the vocal cords. It is important to stress the direct visualization of both the blade and tube past the oral cavity and soft palate as an indirect technique will put the patient at high risk for injury. The options provided by this type of blade allow for greater flexibility in technique for the provider and improved teaching of techniques, with all present having the ability to see what the laryngoscopist views. The video source allows for a supervising provider to see in real time what the performing provider sees, allowing for instruction or assistance on both direct and indirect techniques. For more difficult airways, the ability for multiple clinicians to view the airway can allow for earlier assistance.

As for acute-angle video laryngoscopes, examples of available devices include GlideScope® LoPro, Storz C-mac D-blade, and single-use GlideScope® AVL and McGRATH™ X-blades. These blades are oriented upward at a steeper angle as previously mentioned, allowing for better anterior visualization. For example, the GlideScope® blades are oriented upward at a 60-degree angle. Due to this angulation, these blades cannot be used for direct visualization and require the use of a stylet or tracheal introducer. The technique again begins with proper patient positioning and opening of the mouth in the same fashion as with direct laryngoscopy. The blade however is inserted midline and the tongue is not displaced. The blade is directly visualized until passing the soft palate. At this point, indirect visualizing of the blade into position is required. It is typically unnecessary to advance the blade fully into the vallecula, as deep insertion will rotate the laryngeal axis anteriorly, increasing the difficulty of endotracheal tube insertion. A shallower insertion will allow for a wider visual field, provide a straighter pathway for endotracheal tube delivery, and decrease both the distance from lips to the camera and the area of blind-zone during which the provider cannot see the tube tip. One study demonstrated a deliberately restricted view resulted in faster and easier tracheal intubation with no additional complications [1]. Gently lifting the blade will allow for proper visualization after which the endotracheal tube can be indirectly advanced past the soft palate and then indirectly passed through the vocal cords and removing the stylet prior to full advancement into the trachea.

Channeled blades are shaped to match the anatomic curve of the upper airway and to be positioned around the base of the tongue. This allows for exposure of laryngeal structures while reducing cervical manipulation and not requiring tongue displacement. The endotracheal tube is advanced through the channel and hence a limitation is that it is not possible to independently manipulate the tube. The bulkier design and limited use in patients with small mouth openings are additional disadvantages. Examples of these blades include AIRTRAQ AVANT, Airway Scope (Pentax), and King Vision (Ambu). Typically, these blades are entirely disposable or have single-use components.

3. Advantages and disadvantages of video laryngoscopy

Regardless of the specific blade or type of device utilized, video-assisted laryngoscopy (VL) increases the rate of successful intubation in elective airways, difficult airways, and those of the critically ill patient [2]. Certain devices allow for recording and capturing of images, which are useful again for teaching purposes or storing of various anatomical findings. The VL view can be saved in the patient's record for future clinicians to observe and thereby provide critical clinical documentation that has historically been very much subject to the interpretation of the laryngoscopist. The VL, with its ability for multiple clinicians to simultaneously visualize the airway, has become a critical device for teaching and other settings where additional assistance may be necessary. Simple prior maneuvers, such as the BURP (backward, upward, and rightward pressure), become significantly more effective when the assistant is able to visualize the effects of the movement on the laryngoscopic view.

Because video-laryngoscopes are designed to allow for visualization of structures that are not within a direct line of sight, VL intubations are often of great benefit in patients with altered airway anatomy or suboptimal positioning, as the oral-pharyngeal-largyngeal axes do not need to be aligned for successful intubation. VL may reduce cervical spine motion and allow for lower lift force [3, 4]. It is postulated that VL reduces the stress response to laryngoscopy, though no current studies are available to show significant different hemodynamic differences between VL and DL techniques [5–8].

There are still some opponents of VL technology, though there are fewer now than before due to the improvements in resolution, availability, and clinicians' familiarity with these devices. Arguments against widespread VL use now focus on the cost and time to intubation. The setup of VL is certainly more expensive than DL, with components that may need sterile processing, increasing the yearly cost of airway management. While incidence of successful intubation has been documented, the time to successful intubation, with a maximum apneic limit of 60 seconds, has not been shown to be faster with VL over DL. Thus, the comparative advantage of VL over DL may not be superior. Additionally, the rise in VL use may significantly affect the art and practice of DL, which causes DL technique to suffer.

Videolaryngoscopy is not without potential complication. Reported incidence of videolarynscopy-related otolaryngologic complications is around 1%, with most injuries being minor [9]. Injury most likely with blind introduction of an endotracheal tube through the oropharynx, as the anesthetist is focused on the videolaryngoscope screen. Soft tissue injury may occur at various sites in the aerodigestive tract. While most injuries are minor lacerations, some palate injuries may require intervention by an otolaryngologist. Injuries that are recommended for immediate repair prior to extubation are gaping or perforated injuries with a hanging flap. It is important to evaluate and recognize such injuries in order to prevent potential negative consequences that may include bleeding, infection, retropharyngeal abscess formation, and potentially the inability to safely extubate the patient [10]. Proper training with appropriate visualization during intubation is essential to minimize such soft tissue complications.

4. Video laryngoscopy use guidelines

The 2022 American Society of Anesthesiologists Practice Guidelines for Management of the Difficult Airway defines a difficult laryngoscopy as "not possible to visualize any portion of the vocal cords after multiple attempts at laryngoscopy". Evidence cited in the guidelines support the use of video-assisted laryngoscopy in patients with predicted difficult airways. As stated in the guidelines, meta-analyses of randomized controlled trials comparing video-assisted laryngoscopy with direct laryngoscopy in these patients reported improved laryngeal views, higher frequency of successful intubations, higher frequency of first-attempt intubations, and fewer maneuvers with video-assisted laryngoscopy [4, 11–20]. Differences in time to intubation between the two techniques were equivocal [12, 14–16, 19–22]. When comparing video-assisted laryngoscopy with airway laryngoscopy using a flexible intubation scope, randomized controlled trials reported equivocal findings for laryngeal view, visualization time, first-attempt intubation success, and time to intubation [23–26]. In terms of which video laryngoscope is recommended, when comparing hyper-angulated video laryngoscopes with non-angulated video laryngoscopes for anticipated difficult airways, randomized controlled trials reported equivocal findings for laryngoscopic view, intubation success, first-attempt intubation success, and time to intubation [18, 20]. Additionally, comparisons of channel-guided with non-channel-guided video laryngoscopes found equivocal results for laryngeal view, intubation success, first-attempt intubation, time to intubation, and needed intubation maneuvers [17, 27]. VL is currently considered a first-line airway maneuver in airway management algorithms around the world and is being viewed as essential to standard of care in airway management.

5. Conclusions

As compared with direct laryngoscopy, video-assisted laryngoscopy often improves laryngeal views and increases the frequency of successful intubations. VL has become a very popular technique and is included in the Practice Guidelines of Difficult Airway Management for the American Society of Anesthesiologists, as well as other anesthesia societies world-wide. With the current widespread adoption of this technology, gaining familiarity with the various types of video-laryngoscopes that are now available is critical for any practitioner who is managing a patient's airway.

DOI: http://dx.doi.org/10.5772/intechopen.108176

Conflict of interest

The authors declare no conflict of interest.

Author details

William Pender, Jessica A. Lovich-Sapola* and Kasia P. Rubin
Cleveland Clinic, Cleveland, OH, USA

*Address all correspondence to: jlsapola@gmail.com

References

[1] Gu Y, Robert J, Kovacs G, Milne AD, Morris I, Hung O, et al. A deliberately restricted laryngeal view with the GlideScope® video laryngoscope is associated with faster and easier tracheal intubation when compared with a full glottic view: A randomized clinical trial. Canadian Journal of Anaesthesia. 2016;**63**(8):928-937

[2] Pieters BMA et al. Videolaryngoscopy vs. direct laryngoscopy use by experienced anaesthetists in patients with known difficult airways: A systematic review and meta-analysis. Anaesthesia. 2017;**72**(12):1532-1541

[3] Russell T, Khan S, Elman J, Katznelson R, Cooper RM. Measurement of forces applied during Macintosh direct laryngoscopy compared with GlideScope ® videolaryngoscopy*: Applied forces during videolaryngoscopy. Anaesthesia. 2012;**67**(6):626-631

[4] Cordovani D, Russell T, Wee W, Suen A, Cooper RM. Measurement of forces applied using a Macintosh direct laryngoscope compared with a Glidescope video laryngoscope in patients with predictors of difficult laryngoscopy: A randomised controlled trial. European Journal of Anaesthesiology. 2019;**36**(3):221-226

[5] Xue FS, Zhang GH, Li XY, Sun HT, Li P, Li CW, et al. Comparison of hemodynamic responses to orotracheal intubation with the GlideScope videolaryngoscope and the Macintosh direct laryngoscope. Journal of Clinical Anesthesia. 2007;**19**(4):245-250

[6] Siddiqui N, Katznelson R, Friedman Z. Heart rate/blood pressure response and airway morbidity following tracheal intubation with direct laryngoscopy, GlideScope and Trachlight: A randomized control trial. European Journal of Anaesthesiology. 2009;**26**(9):740-745

[7] Koh JC, Lee JS, Lee YW, Chang CH. Comparison of the laryngeal view during intubation using Airtraq and Macintosh laryngoscopes in patients with cervical spine immobilization and mouth opening limitation. Korean Journal of Anesthesiology. 2010;**59**(5):314-318

[8] Sarkılar G, Sargın M, Sarıtaş TB, Borazan H, Gök F, Kılıçaslan A, et al. Hemodynamic responses to endotracheal intubation performed with video and direct laryngoscopy in patients scheduled for major cardiac surgery. International Journal of Clinical and Experimental Medicine. 2015;**8**(7):11477-11483

[9] Howell JF, Appelbaum EN, Lee TS. Dangers of Videolaryngoscopy-assisted intubation: Risk for multiple Otolaryngologic complications. Surgical Case Reports. 2018;**2**(2):2-3

[10] Greer D, Marshall KE, Bevans S, Standlee A, McAdams P, et al. Review of videolaryngoscopy pharyngeal wall injuries. Laryngoscope. 2017;**127**:349-353

[11] Aziz MF, Dillman D, Fu R, Brambrink AM. Comparative effectiveness of the C-MAC video laryngoscope *versus* direct laryngoscopy in the setting of the predicted difficult airway. Anesthesiology. 2012;**116**(3):629-636

[12] Ali QE, Amir SH, Ahmed S. A comparative evaluation of king vision video laryngoscope (channelled blade), McCoy, and Macintosh laryngoscopes for tracheal intubation in patients with immobilized cervical spine. Sri Lankan Journal of Anaesthesiology. 2017;**25**(2):70

[13] Gupta N, Rath GP, Prabhakar H. Clinical evaluation of C-MAC videolaryngoscope with or without use of stylet for endotracheal intubation in patients with cervical spine immobilization. Journal of Anesthesia. 2013;**27**(5):663-670

[14] Hazarika H, Saxena A, Meshram P, Kumar BA. A randomized controlled trial comparing C mac D blade and Macintosh laryngoscope for nasotracheal intubation in patients undergoing surgeries for head and neck cancer. Saudi Journal of Anaesthesia. 2018;**12**(1):35-41

[15] Jungbauer A, Schumann M, Brunkhorst V, Börgers A, Groeben H. Expected difficult tracheal intubation: A prospective comparison of direct laryngoscopy and video laryngoscopy in 200 patients. British Journal of Anaesthesia. 2009;**102**(4):546-550

[16] Liu L, Yue H, Li J. Comparison of three tracheal intubation techniques in thyroid tumor patients with a difficult airway: A randomized controlled trial. Medical Principles and Practice. 2014;**23**(5):448-452

[17] Malik MA, Subramaniam R, Maharaj CH, Harte BH, Laffey JG. Randomized controlled trial of the Pentax AWS®, Glidescope®, and Macintosh laryngoscopes in predicted difficult intubation. British Journal of Anaesthesia. 2009;**103**(5):761-768

[18] Serocki G, Bein B, Scholz J, Dörges V. Management of the predicted difficult airway: A comparison of conventional blade laryngoscopy with video-assisted blade laryngoscopy and the GlideScope. European Journal of Anaesthesiology. 2010;**27**(1):24-30

[19] Serocki G, Neumann T, Scharf E, Dörges V, Cavus E. Indirect videolaryngoscopy with C-MAC D-blade and GlideScope: A randomized, controlled comparison in patients with suspected difficult airways. Minerva Anestesiologica. 2013;**79**(2):121-129

[20] Zhu H, Liu J, Suo L, Zhou C, Sun Y, Jiang H. A randomized controlled comparison of non-channeled king vision, McGrath MAC video laryngoscope and Macintosh direct laryngoscope for nasotracheal intubation in patients with predicted difficult intubations. BMC Anesthesiology. 2019;**19**(1):166

[21] Okumura Y, Okuda M, Sato Boku A, Tachi N, Hashimoto M, Yamada T, et al. Usefulness of airway scope for intubation of infants with cleft lip and palate–comparison with Macintosh laryngoscope: A randomized controlled trial. BMC Anesthesiology. 2019;**19**(1):12

[22] Pappu A, Sharma B, Jain R, Dua N, Sood J. A randomised comparative study of “videoendoscope” with the Truview EVO2, C-MAC D blade videolaryngoscope and the Macintosh laryngoscope. Indian Journal of Anaesthesia. 2020;**64**(15):186

[23] Abdellatif AA, Ali MA. GlideScope videolaryngoscope versus flexible fiberoptic bronchoscope for awake intubation of morbidly obese patient with predicted difficult intubation. Middle East Journal of Anaesthesiology. 2014;**22**(4):385-392

[24] Nassar M, Zanaty OM, Ibrahim M. Bonfils fiberscope vs GlideScope for awake intubation in morbidly obese patients with expected difficult airways. Journal of Clinical Anesthesia. 2016;**32**:101-105

[25] Rosenstock CV, Thøgersen B, Afshari A, Christensen AL, Eriksen C, Gätke MR. Awake Fiberoptic or awake video Laryngoscopic tracheal intubation

in patients with anticipated difficult airway management. Anesthesiology. 2012;**116**(6):1210-1216

[26] Wahba SS, Tammam TF, Saeed AM. Comparative study of awake endotracheal intubation with Glidescope video laryngoscope versus flexible fiber optic bronchoscope in patients with traumatic cervical spine injury. Egyptian Journal of Anaesthesia. 2012;**28**(4):257-260

[27] Markham TH, Nwokolo OO, Guzman-Reyes S, Medina-Rivera G, Gumbert SD, Cai C, et al. A comparison of the king vision® and glidescope® video intubation systems in patients at risk for difficult intubation. Trends in Anaesthesia and Critical Care. 2019;**28**:27-35

Chapter 3

Ultrasound (US) Imaging Use in the Management of the Difficult Tracheal Intubation

Ajay Singh, Ankita Dhir, Shiv Lal Soni, Rekha Gupta, Naveen B. Naik, Kashish Garg, Venkata Ganesh and Narender Kaloria

Abstract

The ultrasound has been in clinical use since the early 1900s, but its use in the airway has not been published extensively so far. Combining the skills of USG with thorough knowledge of regional anatomy can prove to be a boon to improving the quality of care being delivered to patients. Preoperative use of USG at different levels of the neck combined with the risk assessment methods can help to organize predictors of difficult airway and difficult laryngoscopy. Basic comprehension of USG physics, transducer selection, and probe orientation and a better understanding of airway anatomy contribute to the accuracy of ultrasound interpretation. In day-to-day practice, there is a potential for failed tracheal intubations followed by failure of gaining adequate access to the airway, thus posing challenges to anesthesiologists. Besides predicting difficult airway, USG provides an incentive to properly place an endotracheal tube (ETT) to an adequate depth, estimation of the size of ETT particularly helpful in children and obese, laryngeal mask airway (LMA) confirmation, surgical airways, and post-extubation stridor assessment and thus prevents the risk of reintubation. With the promising and increasing number of evidence exists, there is potential for incorporation of upper airway USG into further standard of care assessment, monitoring, and imaging modalities.

Keywords: airway, predictors, ultrasonography, ultrasound imaging, tracheal intubation

1. Introduction

The difficult airway has been defined as "the clinical situation in which a conventionally trained anesthesiologist experiences difficulty with face mask ventilation or difficulty with tracheal intubation or both." Failure to assess or identify a difficult airway and not make an organized plan for the management of the airway may lead to a poor outcome. Assessment of the airway goes beyond bedside clinical tests and should emphasize the identification of problems during each step of airway management [1]. This should involve the proper assessment of variations in anatomy, various airway pathologies, and the previous approach used in prior cases. These variable factors play decisive role in determining the success of any equipment or technique or adjunct used and most importantly incorporate the skill and knowledge of anesthetist about various techniques and equipment.

2. Incidence

The incidence of difficult airway can range between 5.8 and 20% according to previous studies [2–5]. This high incidence is probably because of various definitions of difficult airway either using the Intubation Difficulty Scale or the modified mallampati (MMP) grading. None of these studies, however, have reported ultrasound measures consistently.

3. Assessment of difficult airway

3.1 Clinical history

It is important to start by reviewing the previous medical records regarding airway management and whether there was any difficulty faced and how it was handled. It can be very informational to communicate with the previous anesthesia team regarding the airway management, if their anesthesia chart reflected any difficulty. Proper documentation of the airway management is important, including techniques that were and were not successful. All of this is of value if there is no worsening or new-onset airway pathologies. This information should be recorded in all cases irrespective of difficult airway for the benefit of future colleagues.

In your preoperative examination, there are many medical conditions that have been associated with an increased risk of difficult intubation and airway management. In progressive disorders such as chronic rheumatoid arthritis, chronic ankylosing spondylitis, and chronic diabetes mellitus, disease involvement of the airway or neck joints should be ruled out. Rare syndromes such as Pierre-Robin syndrome, Klippel-Feil syndrome, and Treacher Collins syndrome are often associated with difficult airways. History of recent acute respiratory tract infections has increased incidence of laryngospasm and bronchospasm especially in children.

A STOPBANG questionnaire should answered by all patients prior to anesthesia, to assess the potential risk for obstructive sleep apnea (OSA). Patients with diagnosed OSA are at increased risk for difficult airway management.

Any new-onset airway pathology or worsening pathology must be documented as it will require entirely different approach to manage.

Patients presenting with a retrosternal goiter should be evaluated for signs and symptoms suggestive of tracheal compression or recurrent laryngeal nerve compression such as the degree of hoarseness or voice change and its progression and stridor. Also underlying esophageal compression resulting in drooling of secretions, dysphagia, and ability to lie supine should be documented. It should also be documented in what position symptoms are relieved.

The trauma patient with any airway injury requires a thorough evaluation. Assessment should focus on the swelling and its onset, associated pain and trismus, and time since injury. In case of chemical and thermal burns, careful assessment should be done as mucosal edema can develop rapidly and progress very fast. Difficult airway is 10 times more commonly encountered in intensive care unit and emergency area [6].

3.2 Clinical assessment

The airway assessment should start with direct observation for obesity, bearded face, pregnancy, prominent breasts, and visible external signs of head and neck disease such as large thyroid mass or Ludwigs angina. There are specific tests to predict a difficult airway; however, there is no ideal airway assessment tool due to lack of statistical predictive power of individual airway tests. These tests, however, should alert us for the potential of a difficult airway so that appropriate measures can be taken beforehand for patient safety.

3.2.1 Clinical airway examination

- Inter-incisor distance commonly measured by mouth opening: Less than 3 cm distance is usually taken as non-reassuring sign. However, some supraglottic airway devices (SADs) such as supreme laryngeal mask airway (LMA) require <2 cm mouth opening and certain videolaryngoscope (VL) blades require barely 1.8 to 2 cm for laryngoscope insertion.

- The modified mallampati (MMP) classification: MMP is used to assess the ratio of the tongue size with oropharyngeal cavity size. The patient is examined in the sitting position, with their mouth wide open and maximal tongue protrusion. It scores from 1 to 4 based on the anatomy. Class 3 MMP (soft palate and base of uvula visible) and Class 4 MMP (only hard palate visible) are indicators of difficult mask ventilation (DMV) and difficult laryngoscopy (DL); however, they are associated with poor positive predictive value (PPV) and inter-observer reliability if used alone.

- Patil test, also known as thyromental distance (TMD): measured from the upper border of thyroid cartilage to lower border of jaw with the head extended. TMD of <6.5 cm is considered an increased risk for difficult laryngoscopy.

- Sterno-mental distance (SMD), known as Sava test: measured from the notch of the manubrium sterni to the lower border of mandible with the head in extension position. Less than 12.5 cm of SMD has been associated with a difficult laryngoscopy. For measuring these distances, use of ruler or measuring tape is better than fingerbreadths as they are more reliable and accurate.

- The neck circumference to TMD ratio of more than 5.0 is considered as an improved predictor of a difficult airway. The ratio of patient height to TMD, known as RHTMD, is also said to be a good predictor of difficult airway [7].

- To assess temporomandibular joint function, upper lip bite test and jaw protrusion are done. It takes into account prognathic ability of temporomandibular joint and prominence of maxillary teeth. Attention should be given to dentition, loose teeth, artificial dentures, and single maxillary incisors.

- Range of neck movements should be assessed to ensure whether the patient is able to do the classic "sniffing position" (flexion at cervical spine and extension at atlanto-occipital joint) for adequate mask ventilation and laryngoscopy along with proper position for tracheostomy, if required in an emergency.

- The cricothyroid membrane should also be identified in a patient with a potential difficult airway, in case of an emergent need to do a cricothyrotomy.

- Assessment of submandibular space is also useful as compliance of tissue alters due to neck infection, irradiation, or burns, and this can result in difficulty in tongue displacement into the submandibular space during laryngoscopy [8].

- Tissue compliance can be examined by tongue protrusion by patient. Decreased tongue mobility demonstrates decreased compliance.

3.3 Predictors of difficult mask ventilation (DMV)

The incidence of DMV ranges between 5 and 5.8% of all general anesthetics [9]. There are several predictors for DMV.

- One of the mnemonics that can be used to evaluate for a potential DMV is OBESE (Obesity, Beard, Elderly (>55 year), history of snoring, and edentulous mouth).

- Modified mallampati class 3 or 4, limited jaw protrusion, and male sex are the important risk factors.

- History of neck irradiation is an important predictor of impossible mask ventilation situation, defined as ineffective patient ventilation despite usage of various adjuncts, neuromuscular blockade, and multiple healthcare providers. This occurs because neck irradiation causes noncompliant tissue fibrosis involving the airway. Obesity and BMI both are not useful predictors; however, they are marker for increased aspiration risk and poor oxygen reserve due to reduced functional residual capacity. The real body fat distribution is important to predict a difficult airway. Airway collapsibility is increased by fat deposition in the parapharyngeal tissues, which predisposes to OSA [8]. This pattern is more commonly seen in male pattern obesity where fat is more often deposited around neck and upper torso. The increased fat deposition around neck can cause airway narrowing.

3.4 Predicting difficulty in airway instrumentation

Assessment of the nasal passages should be done for nasopharyngeal airway insertion in case of nasal intubation, upper airway obstruction, or failing airway management as a rescue adjunct. Nasotracheal instrumentation can lead to trauma and epistaxis. So prior doing this, patency of nostrils, any presence of septal deviation, polyps, etc., should be looked for to avoid complications and increasing overall difficulty. Presence of clotting disorders or basal skull fractures should be warranted prior to nasal instrumentation.

Restricted mouth opening limits the insertion of almost all devices. So inter-incisor gap should be assessed so that appropriate oral devices can be used electively or in emergency situation. SADs and thin VL blades require mouth opening of < 3 cm, whereas Macintosh blade requires 3 cm inter-incisor gap. In patients with restricted mouth opening, the anesthesia team should have full knowledge of the pros and cons of the VL devices over the fiber optic technique. A high arched or narrow palate can reduce blade space in the oropharynx. Large breasts and barrel chests can pose difficult laryngoscope insertion; however, "ramp" position and appropriate device selection such as polio blade come as rescue. Indirect laryngoscopy can be fruitful in cases with relative or absolute retrognathia and restricted neck extension [10]. Cricoid pressure is an important part of rapid sequence induction; however, it can reduce optimal glottis visualization; however, in case of a difficult airway or difficult SAD insertion, cricoid pressure can be withdrawn under direct vision for improved glottis visualization or ease of SAD insertion, respectively.

Surgical airway such as cricothyrotomy or emergency tracheostomy are kept as a rescue in "can't intubate, can't ventilate" (CICV) situation. In patients with complex head and neck surgery or in anticipated emergency airway obstruction, the surgical airway is kept as rescue technique during the induction of anesthesia [8]. A difficult airway is anticipated in patients having history of neck radiation, obesity with fat deposited around anterior neck, thyroid mass or neck mass with or without deviation of trachea, previous tracheostomy, short neck, restricted neck flexion, and extension deformities. It is difficult to identify anatomical landmarks in young children and female patients. So in these patients with anticipated difficulty, anatomical landmarks should be marked with ultrasound assistance preoperatively.

3.5 Predictors of difficult laryngoscopy

A traumatic laryngoscopy can result in failure to secure the airway or unanticipated difficulty. The first attempt should always be the best attempt, particularly in cases of difficult airway so that strategies can be formulated with best available facilities.

Anatomical factors such as prominent incisors, retrognathia, macroglossia, and small inter-incisor gap affect insertion of the laryngoscope and alter the final view achieved by line of sight approach [8]. Short TMD and SMD are the indicators of an anterior larynx relative to line of sight. Due to in proportionate tongue and oral cavity relationship, modified mallampati class 3 or 4 are the good predictors of DL. Limited neck extension because of increased pretracheal tissue, large occiput, or large neck circumference has been associated with a difficult airway as it causes difficulty to achieve sniffing positioning [10]. Diseases such as lingual tonsil hyperplasia, epiglottitis, and Ludwig's angina are the important predictors of difficult or impossible laryngoscopy.

There are several factors predicting compliance and volume of submandibular tissue such as TMD, temporomandibular joint dysfunction, difficulty in mandibular protrusion, relative tongue volume, and retrognathia. These factors alter tongue displacement into submandibular tissue during laryngoscopy influencing the glottis visualization. Disease affecting the airway such as tumor or pharyngeal adipose tissue deposits also makes the laryngoscopy difficult [10].

3.6 Predictors of difficult intubation

A reduced oropharyngeal space may lead to difficult endotracheal tube manipulation. Endotracheal tube (ETT) size and suitability for awake fiberoptic technique should be assessed for specific pathologies such as vocal cord palsy, laryngeal tumors, and subglottic stenosis [8]. Stridor with or without respiratory distress is an important symptom of these pathologies and should alert the anesthetist. Whether any further investigations are required depend on the onset of stridor and its progression and association with respiratory distress.

3.7 Predicting a difficult extubation

Extubation is extremely important in the airway management. In 2012, The Difficult Airway Society has published extubation guidelines highlighting extubation as an important step in patient management. Laryngeal edema causing airway obstruction is the most common cause of early postoperative reintubation. Many factors influence postoperative airway management and includes traumatic intubation, effects of residual general anesthetic drugs, opioids, inadequate reversal of muscle relaxants, or local anesthetized airway. The residual effect of these agents on respiratory drive and airway reflexes should be ruled out [11]. There are more chances of early desaturation and postoperative airway complications in patients having obesity. Patients undergoing head and neck surgery, airway surgery, having Trendelenburg or prone positions, and prolonged intubation should be assessed carefully prior to extubation.

4. Role of ultrasonography in the upper airway evaluation

Point of care ultrasonography (US) has emerged as a novel, simple, portable, noninvasive tool that can be used for airway assessment and management. It plays a pivotal role in the quick assessment of the airway anatomy in emergency areas and the operation room. With the help of US, upper airway imaging can be used for subglottic stenosis detection, prediction of difficult intubation, verification of ETT placement, percutaneous tracheostomy, cricothyroidotomy, post-extubation stridor evaluation, and preoperative determination of pediatric ETT size and double-lumen endobronchial tube (DLT) size [11].

The basic principle behind US image formation by rarefaction needs to be understood clearly for better interpretation of images. Knowledge of US transducer types and its orientation and relevant airway anatomy are important for proper evaluation.

5. Patient position for ultrasound airway assessment

Optimal supine sniffing position is achieved by placing a pillow under the occiput to achieve optimal neck flexion and head extension. The presence of air makes it difficult to visualize deeper structures because of poor medium. Comet tail and reverberation artifacts are produced by intraluminal air [8]. Bone structures such as ramus of mandible, mentum, hyoid bone, and sternum appear as bright hyperechoic linear structures with a hypoechoic acoustic shadow beneath it. Cartilaginous structures such as thyroid and cricoid cartilages appear as homogeneous hypoechoic [10]. Muscle and connective tissues appear as heterogeneous striated and hypoechoic. Fat and glandular structures appear as homogeneous and mildly to strongly hyperechoic when compared with adjacent soft tissues, depending on the fat content. Air-mucosa (A-M) interface appears as bright hyperechoic linear structure.

6. Applications of ultrasound in airway evaluation

6.1 Ultrasound-guided assessment of the subglottic upper airway diameter and prediction of endotracheal tube size

US has emerged as a reliable tool for assessing the narrowest diameter of the cricoid lumen (transverse diameter). In third decade of life, calcification of the laryngeal cartilages begins to occur because of age factor which creates an acoustic shadow. This limits the use of US in older patients. US-guided subglottic airway diameter measurement is a better indicator of appropriate size of cuffed and uncuffed ETT in pediatric patients.

6.2 Ultrasound measured tongue thickness and difficult intubation

Tongue thickness, measured by US, (**Figure 1**) greater than 6.1 cm, has been shown to be an independent predictor of difficult intubation with 75% sensitivity and 72% specificity. A ratio of tongue thickness to thyromental distance greater than 0.87 has an 84% sensitivity and 79% specificity for predicting difficult tracheal intubation [12].

6.3 Ultrasound-guided prediction of difficult laryngoscopy in the obese patient

US-guided anterior neck soft tissue thickness measurement predicts difficult laryngoscopy. The measurement is done from skin to the anterior aspect of trachea at three levels: vocal cord, thyroid isthmus, and suprasternal notch. Soft tissue thickness at the vocal cords level is a better predictor of difficult laryngoscopy in obese patients. Soft tissue at each level can be calculated by averaging the soft tissue thickness in millimeters obtained in the central axis of the neck and 15 mm to the left and right pretracheal soft tissue. Patients having neck circumference of 50 cm

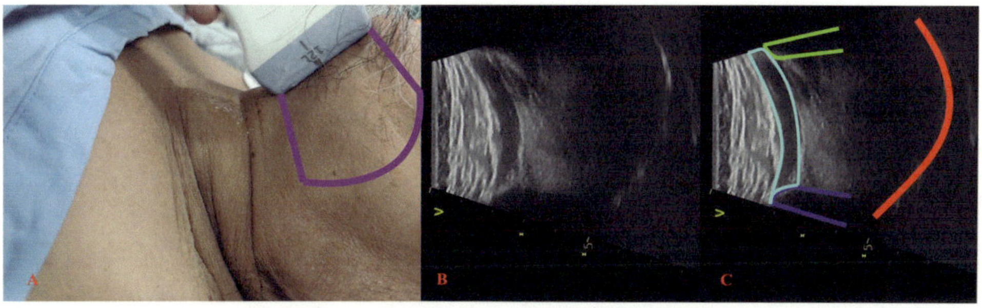

Figure 1.
*(A) Photograph showing probe placement and zone of insonation (area within purple boundary); **(B & C)** ultrasound image showing mylohyoid (sky blue), mandible (green), hyoid (dark blue), and dorsal surface of tongue (red). (image credits: Author Dr Venkata Ganesh).*

and pretracheal soft tissue thickness of 28 mm at vocal cords level have difficulty while doing laryngoscopy [13].

6.4 Ultrasound-guided prediction of post-extubation stridor

In intubated patients, assessment of vocal cords and larynx morphology by US helps to predict post-extubation stridor. US-guided air-column width measurement identifies patients at higher risk for post-extubation stridor so that appropriate measures can be taken after extubation. A reduced laryngeal air column width difference or ratio (pre-intubation vs. pre-extubation values, with the ETT cuff deflated) has been shown to be a good predictor of post-extubation stridor [14, 15]. **Figure 2** demonstrates measurement of air column width with the cuff deflated.

6.5 Ultrasound-guided emergency cricothyrotomy and elective transtracheal cannulation

For securing surgical airways, identification of the exact location of the trachea is very important to manage the difficult airway in both elective and emergency scenario. With the help of US, the trachea can be visualized before both emergency cricothyrotomy and elective transtracheal cannulation. A visual guide to identify airway-related structures is presented in **Figures 3** and **4**. This is useful in anticipated difficult airway such as neck swelling, thyroid mass, and Ludwig's angina where localization of trachea is difficult.

6.6 Ultrasound-guided airway blocks to facilitate awake intubation

For performing upper airway blocks in fiberoptic bronchoscopy, US plays an important role. It helps to identify superior laryngeal nerve (SLN) for SLN block. SLN running between thyroid cartilage and hyoid bone can be easily seen on transverse US

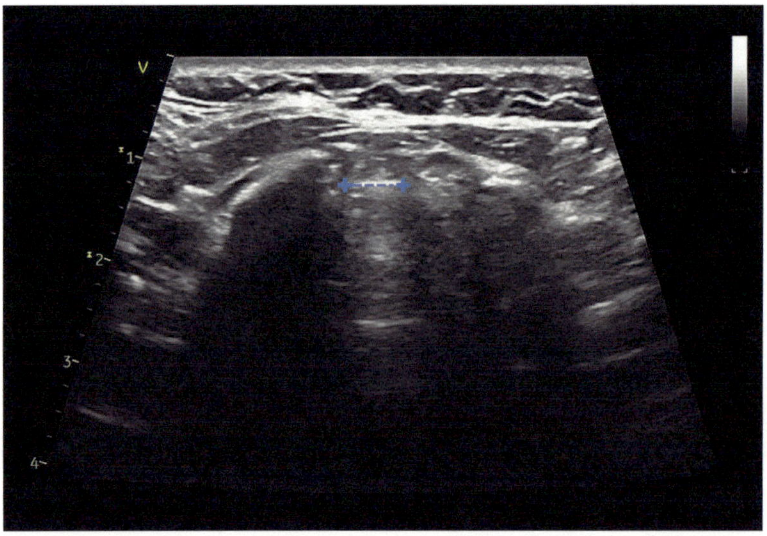

Figure 2.
Measurement of laryngeal air column (US probe placed transverse across the trachea). The length of the blue dashed/discontinuous line is the width of the air column (image credits: Author Dr Venkata Ganesh).

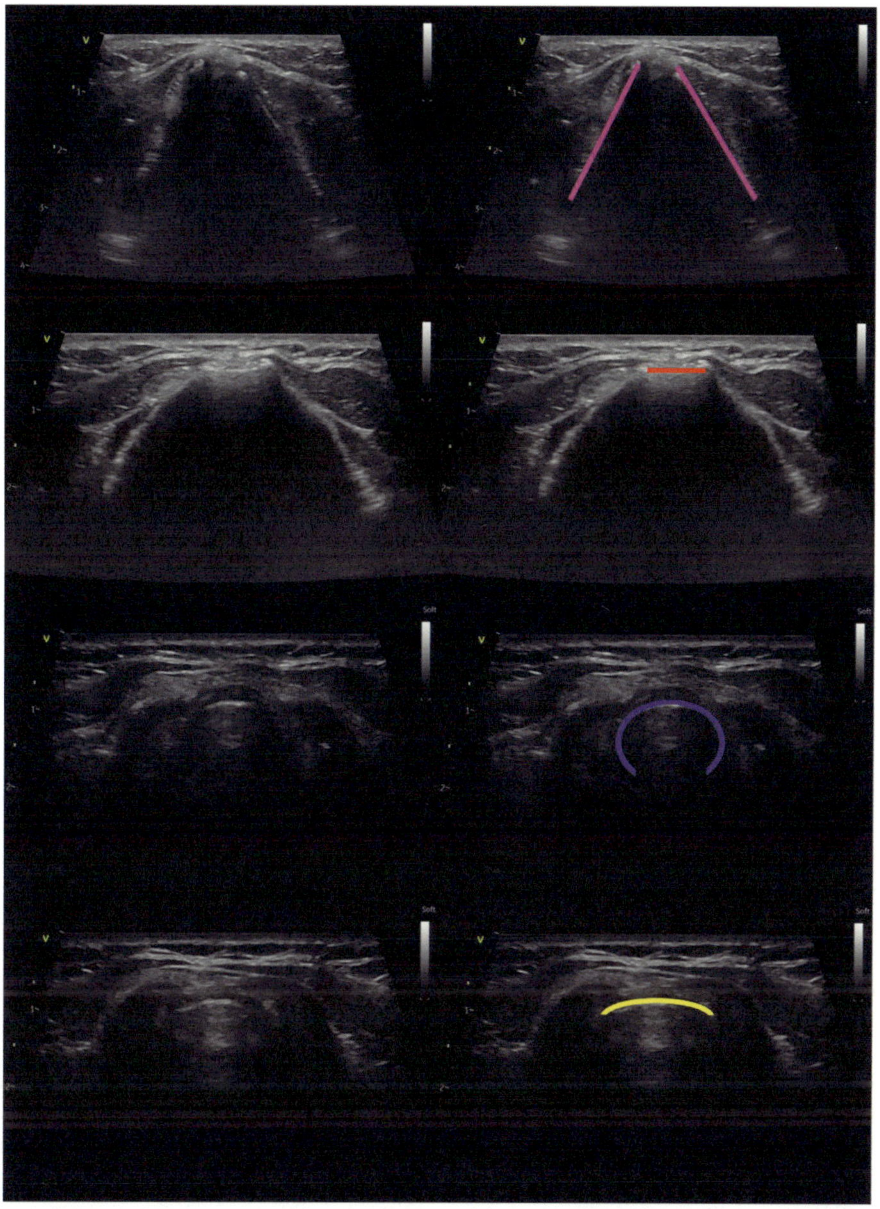

Figure 3.
With the US probe placed in the transverse plane and scanning cephalocaudally, the topmost image shows the thyroid cartilage (magenta) followed caudally by the cricothyroid membrane (red), cricoid (dark blue), and the trachea (yellow). (image credits: Author Dr Venkata Ganesh).

at hyoid bone level. The membrane between the thyroid cartilage and hyoid bone is an iso-echoic line from both sides of the hyoid bone with hyperechoic air below [16].

6.7 Ultrasound-guided intubation

Endotracheal intubation is conventionally confirmed by capnography, five point chest auscultation, and esophageal intubating devices. US-guided equal movement

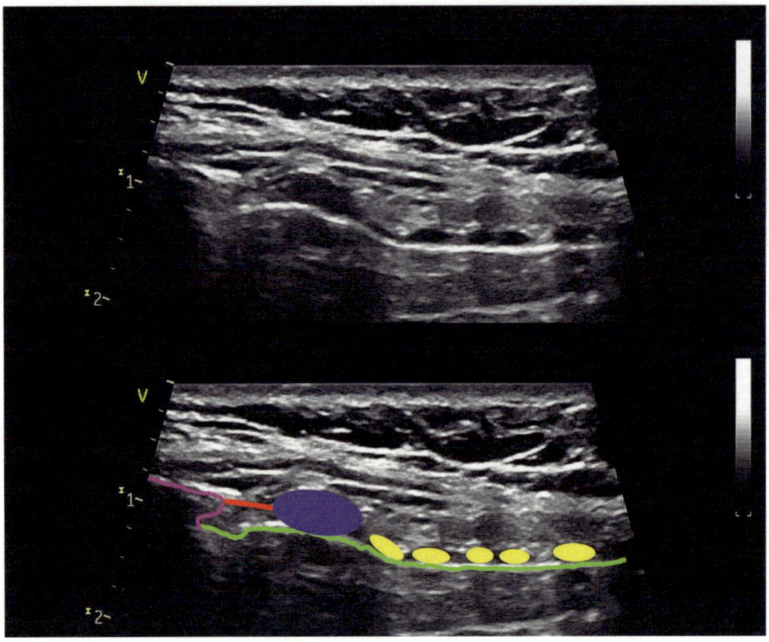

Figure 4.
String of pearls appearance (US probe placed in the saggital plane). Magenta—thyroid cartilage; red—cricothyroid membrane; dark blue—cricoid; yellow—trachea. (image credits: Author Dr Venkata Ganesh).

of bilateral pleura and diaphragm indicating expansion of lungs is an indirect sign of correct physiological function of the tracheal tube in mechanically ventilated patients. Lung sliding sign seen on intercostal US view at interface of lung-chest wall also indicates lung expansion.

Esophageal intubation can be identified if the esophagus is lateral to the trachea (**Figure 5**). When intubating under real-time ultrasound guidance, the lack of a disruption in the tracheal air column with a noticeable movement in the esophagus can detect esophageal intubations earlier than capnography or auscultation [17] *(image credits: Author Dr Venkata Ganesh).*

Esophageal intubation results in a paradoxical or immobile state of the diaphragm. Esophageal intubation causes paradoxical ventilation where the diaphragm moves toward the chest due to raised intra-abdominal pressure caused by stomach distension by positive pressure ventilation.

US can also be used to diagnose endobronchial intubation by assessing the diaphragm movement and lung-slide sign on the ventilated lung side (endobronchial) and absent or restricted diaphragm movement and absent lung-slide sign on the non-ventilated lung side [13].

Normal pediatric airway can be visualized in real time using US during tracheal intubation by assessing 1) trachea and tracheal rings identification, 2) vocal cords visualization, 3) widening of glottis with passage of ETT, and 4) confirmation of ETT position above the carina and visualization of sliding sign after manual lung ventilation.

6.8 Ultrasound-guided prediction of left-sided DLT size

Outer tracheal ring diameter is a useful predictor of left main bronchus diameter on ultrasonography and hence helps in selecting left-sided DLT.

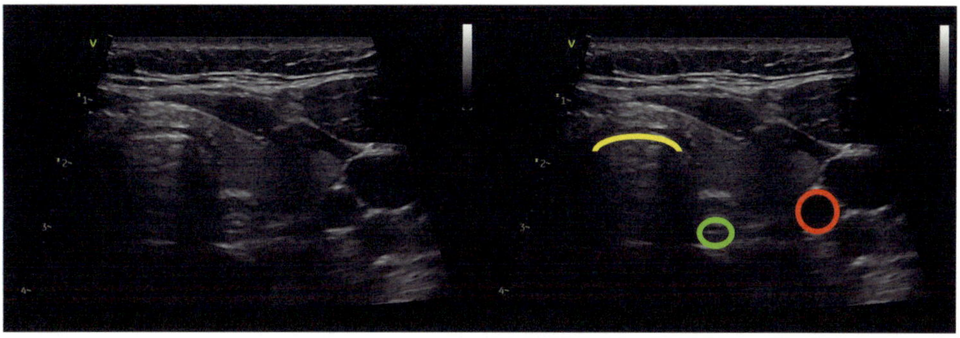

Figure 5.
US image showing trachea (yellow), esophagus to its right (green) and the carotid (red). (image credits: Author Dr Venkata Ganesh).

6.9 Ultrasound-guided detection of laryngeal mask airway position

With the help of US, position of the LMA cuff can be confirmed. For adequate ventilation, the LMA cuff should be placed at the proper position to seal the larynx. LMA should be repositioned if it is not visualized equally on both sides of the larynx on ultrasound [18].

6.10 Ultrasound-guided diagnosis of upper airway pathologies

The US can be used to assess and diagnose upper airway inflammatory diseases such as epiglottitis and mucosal swelling. It can also be used to assess vocal cord mobility. Before securing nasal intubation, maxillary sinusitis or basal skull fractures should be ruled out. Maxillary sinusitis can be diagnosed by US. Boundaries of the maxillary sinus are orbital floor superiorly, hard palate inferiorly, nasal wall medially, and zygoma laterally. Sinus is normally air filled and thus impairs ultrasonic beam transmission. Only the anterior wall is seen with some artifact (acoustic shadowing), which obscures all of the underlying structures. If the sinus is filled with fluid, the ultrasonic beam will travel through the fluid after penetrating the anterior wall and gets reflected by the posterior or lateral walls producing an image known as "sinusogram." In the case of air-fluid level in the sinus or mucosal thickening, partial sinusogram (only posterior wall or side wall seen) is seen. For this, patient should be in upright position or semi-recumbent position so that fluid (if present) flows according to gravity covering the floor of the sinus and coming in contact with anterior wall.

6.11 Ultrasound-assisted percutaneous dilatational tracheostomy

Many serious complications of percutaneous dilational tracheostomy like hemorrhage, high mediastinal vessels erosion, tracheal stenosis, esophageal disruption, and thyroid isthmus injury can be avoided by precise identification of anterior neck structures with the help of US [16]. Before attempting this, the neck should be examined for a midline trachea, the level of the tracheal ring, thyroid isthmus, vulnerable thyroid vessels, and diameter and the midline location of anterior jugular veins or other aberrant vasculature [18]. With advanced US technology, it will be possible in the future to have the real-time guidance in the placement of dilators and tracheostomy tubes.

7. Conclusion

As reviewed earlier, the use of ultrasound during airway management can help identify anatomical anomalies in the airway structures and the location of cricothyroid membrane (useful in cricothyrotomies) as real-time visual confirmation of endotracheal tube position. Ultrasound measurements can also help in the prediction of difficult mask ventilation and intubation. In addition, lung ultrasound can also help detect pneumothorax which can happen due to barotrauma (during ventilation or tracheostomy) as well as unilateral intubations. The use of ultrasound as a teaching aid during airway management can promote visual learning.

Author details

Ajay Singh*, Ankita Dhir, Shiv Lal Soni, Rekha Gupta, Naveen B. Naik, Kashish Garg, Venkata Ganesh and Narender Kaloria
Department of Anaesthesia and Intensive Care, Post Graduate Institute of Medical Education and Research, Chandigarh, India

*Address all correspondence to: ajay.ydv2509@gmail.com

References

[1] Singh M, Chin KJ, Chan VWS, Wong DT, Prasad GA, Yu E. Use of sonography for airway assessment: An observational study. Journal of Ultrasound Medical Official Journal. 2010;**29**(1):79-85

[2] Koh W, Kim H, Kim K, Ro YJ, Yang HS. Encountering unexpected difficult airway: Relationship with the intubation difficulty scale. Korean Journal of Anesthesiology. 2016;**69**(3):244-249

[3] Adnet F, Racine SX, Borron SW, Clemessy JL, Fournier JL, Lapostolle F, et al. A survey of tracheal intubation difficulty in the operating room: A prospective observational study. Acta Anaesthesiologica Scandinavica. 2001;**45**(3):327-332

[4] Maharaj CH, Buckley E, Harte BH, Laffey JG. Endotracheal intubation in patients with cervical spine immobilization: A comparison of macintosh and airtraq laryngoscopes. Anesthesiology. 2007;**107**(1):53-59

[5] Seo SH, Lee JG, Yu SB, Kim DS, Ryu SJ, Kim KH. Predictors of difficult intubation defined by the intubation difficulty scale (IDS): Predictive value of 7 airway assessment factors. Korean Journal of Anesthesiology. 2012;**63**(6):491-497

[6] Sustić A, Kovac D, Zgaljardić Z, Zupan Z, Krstulović B. Ultrasound-guided percutaneous dilatational tracheostomy: A safe method to avoid cranial misplacement of the tracheostomy tube. Intensive Care Medicine. 2000;**26**(9):1379-1381

[7] Kaniyil S, Anandan K, Thomas S. Ratio of height to thyromental distance as a predictor of difficult laryngoscopy: A prospective observational study. Journal of Anaesthesiology Clinical Pharmacology. 2018;**34**(4):485-489

[8] Ezri T, Gewürtz G, Sessler DI, Medalion B, Szmuk P, Hagberg C, et al. Prediction of difficult laryngoscopy in obese patients by ultrasound quantification of anterior neck soft tissue. Anaesthesia. 2003;**58**(11):1111-1114

[9] Kheterpal S, Healy D, Aziz MF, Shanks AM, Freundlich RE, Linton F, et al. Incidence, predictors, and outcome of difficult mask ventilation combined with difficult laryngoscopy: A report from the multicenter perioperative outcomes group. Anesthesiology. 2013;**119**(6):1360-1369

[10] Shibasaki M, Nakajima Y, Ishii S, Shimizu F, Shime N, Sessler DI. Prediction of pediatric endotracheal tube size by ultrasonography. Anesthesiology. 2010;**113**(4):819-824

[11] Osman A, Sum KM. Role of upper airway ultrasound in airway management. Journal of Intensive Care. 2016;**4**(1):52

[12] Yao W, Wang B. Can tongue thickness measured by ultrasonography predict difficult tracheal intubation? BJA British Journal of Anaesthiology. 2017;**118**(4):601-609

[13] Adhikari S, Zeger W, Schmier C, Crum T, Craven A, Frrokaj I, et al. Pilot study to determine the utility of point-of-care ultrasound in the assessment of difficult laryngoscopy. Academic Emergency Medicine. 2011;**18**(7):754-758

[14] El Amrousy D, Elkashlan M, Elshmaa N, Ragab A. Ultrasound-guided

laryngeal air column width difference as a new predictor for postextubation stridor in children. Critical Care Medicine. 2018;**46**(6):e496

[15] Venkategowda PM, Mahendrakar K, Rao SM, Mutkule DP, Shirodkar CG, Yogesh H. Laryngeal air column width ratio in predicting post extubation stridor. Indian Journal of Critical Care Medicine. 2015;**19**(3):170-173

[16] Kim J, Kim JY, Kim WO, Kil HK. An ultrasound evaluation of laryngeal mask airway position in pediatric patients: An observational study. Anesthesia and Analgesia. 2015;**120**(2):427-432

[17] Chowdhury AR, Punj J, Pandey R, Darlong V, Sinha R, Bhoi D. Ultrasound is a reliable and faster tool for confirmation of endotracheal intubation compared to chest auscultation and capnography when performed by novice anaesthesia residents – A prospective controlled clinical trial. Saudi Journal of Anaesthesia. 2020;**14**(1):15-21

[18] Kajekar P, Mendonca C, Gaur V. Role of ultrasound in airway assessment and management. International Journal of Ultrasound and Applied Technologies in Perioperative Care. 2010;**1**(2):97-100

Chapter 4

A Paradigm Shift of Airway Management: The Role of Video-Assisted Intubating Stylet Technique

Hsiang-Ning Luk, Hsuan-Nu Luk, Jason Zhensheng Qu and Alan Shikani

Abstract

Difficult or failed intubation is a major contributor to morbidity for patients and to liability for the provider. Research to improve understanding, prevention, and management of such complications remains an anesthetic priority, and a driving force behind continuous improvements in intubation techniques and intubation equipment. The purpose of this review article is to focus on the video-assisted intubating stylet technique (VS; also known as the Shikani optical stylet technique for intubation) and video-assisted optical stylet devices, both for routine use and alternative rescue application for tracheal intubation, and stress their advantages as compared to conventional direct laryngoscopy and videolaryngoscopy. The VS technique was introduced by Dr. Alan Shikani in 1996 and popularized with the advent of the Shikani optical stylet and subsequent similar stylets variations. We focus on the clinical details of the technique itself, and on the various advantages and troubleshooting under different clinical scenarios and practice settings. In our experience, video-assisted intubating stylet technique often constitutes the most appropriate approach both for daily routine and emergency airway management. Furthermore, we also emphasize the importance of video-assisted intubating stylets in enhancing the practitioner systems response when difficult or failed tracheal intubation is encountered.

Keywords: airway management, endotracheal intubation, difficult airway, resuscitation, laryngoscopy, video-assisted intubating stylet, Shikani stylet, anesthesia, COVID-19, critical care

1. Introduction

Airway management has often presented challenges for clinicians since the early times when direct laryngoscope (DL) was invented [1, 2]. The complications related to difficult airway or failed tracheal intubation can be devastating to both the patients and the anesthesiologists. Clinicians have continually strived to improve tracheal intubation techniques and devices to avoid complications. In this article, we review the role of video-assisted intubating stylet (VS; also known as the Shikani optical stylet technique for intubation), and we focus on its technical aspects and its potential advantages over conventional DL and videolaryngoscope (VL).

The term "optical stylet" was coined by George Berci and Ronald Katz in 1979 [3, 4]. The main part of this device included a straight rigid endoscope functioning as an endotracheal tube stylet to facilitate endotracheal intubation. The straight design of the stylet was however not workable for cases of difficult laryngoscopy and the device had to be introduced with the aid of a Macintosh laryngoscope. The technique of tracheal intubation with the rigid stylets was later improved in 1983 by Pierre Bonfils with a device that was similar. Instead of a straight design, it employed a fixed curved distal tip at the angle of 40 degrees [5]. This allowed better access to the anteriorly located larynx. In 1996, Alan Shikani introduced the Shikani optical stylet (Clarus Medical, Minneapolis, MN, USA) and the first series were published in 1999 [6], with numerous large studies to follow. The Shikani stylet is semi-malleable and its tip may be bent to better fit to the patient's upper airway anatomy. With this newly designed stylet, Shikani also introduced a technique for tracheal intubation (the Shikani technique). Briefly, the operator grasps patient's mandible with one hand and lifts the jaw anteriorly and then introduces the optical stylet, preloaded with the endotracheal tube with the other hand and advances the combination into the larynx. Because the stylet "sees" where the endotracheal tube is going, successful entry into the trachea is confirmed by direct visualization, and importantly this is done without any need for using a Macintosh blade or putting any pressure on the teeth or extending the cervical spine. The Shikani technique for intubation is described in **Figures 1** and 2.

Figure 3 shows clinical endoscopic views confirming by endoscopy (**Figure 3A**), whereby VS provides clear glottic view before sliding the endotracheal tube (ET tube) into the trachea (**Figure 3B**). VS is superior to DL and VL in obtaining an easy look at the glottic area and ensuring smooth railroading of the ET tube into trachea. Although VL with different angles/shapes of the blades frequently provides a decent laryngeal and glottis view, the operator may sometimes encounter difficulty in sliding the ET tube into the glottis, with occasional laryngeal trauma or misguided esophageal intubation. This could be due to the inherent design of VL device, inadequate mouth opening and/or oropharyngeal space, three axes alignment, etc. [7–11]. These issues are easily circumvented with VS.

Our experience and that of many others has shown optical stylets to be simple, durable, portable and lightweight, easy to learn and handle, affordable, and convenient to clean and disinfect [12–15]. The Clarus Video System (Clarus Medical LLC, Minneapolis, MN, USA) is a modification of the Shikani optical stylet which was originally introduced in the mid 1990s and since then multiple similar video-assisted intubating stylets have also been brought to market (**Table 1**). At our institution, we are currently equipped with 22 sets of four different brands of VS for routine use on daily basis since 2009 (**Figure 4**). Ours is an 1110-bed tertiary medical center with 1788 personnel, 20 operation rooms, 18 attending anesthesiologists, and 54 nurse anesthetists. Out of all surgeries that needed general anesthesia and tracheal intubation, more than 90% of the intubations were performed using VS (**Table 2**). The rest of tracheal intubations were conducted using flexible fiberoptic endoscope (FOB) mostly in some selected predictable difficult airway scenarios. In contrast, VL was

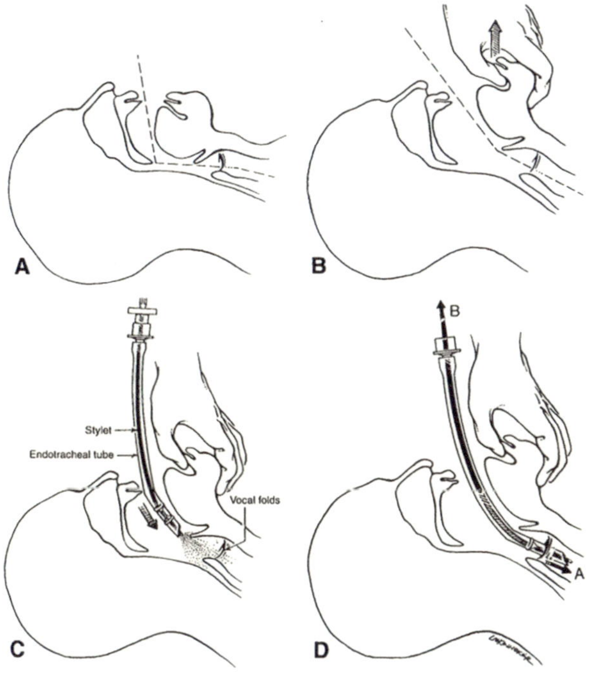

Figure 1.
The Shikani technique for intubation using the Shikani optical stylet. (A) Head is initially in the resting position. (B) Head is placed in the sniffing position, and the mandible is lifted with the left hand. (C) Stylet, preloaded with the endotracheal tube, is inserted into the mouth with the right hand, and the larynx is visualized. (D) Stylet–endotracheal tube unit is advanced through the vocal cords (arrow A) under direct visualization, and the stylet is removed (arrow B). (Courtesy of the SAGE Publishing. Permission to reproduce the images from [6] was granted).

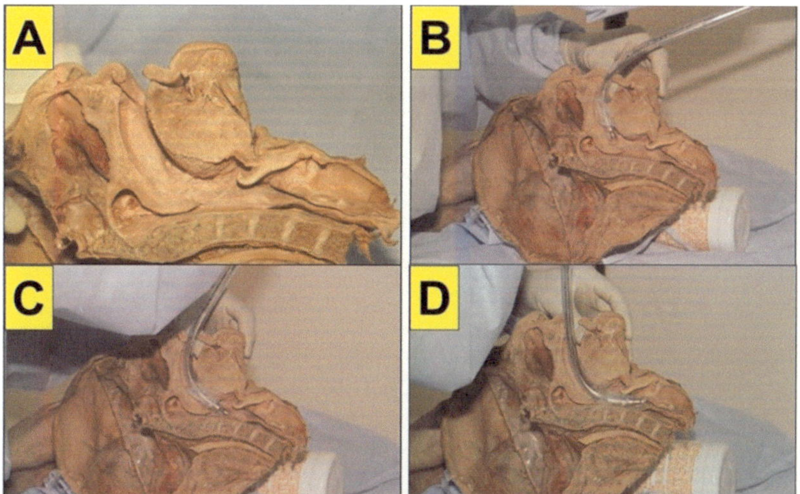

Figure 2.
Demonstration of the Shikani technique for intubation using the Shikani optical stylet in cadavers. (A) Before insertion of VS. The oral space is occupied by the tongue. (B and C) Jaw-thrust by operator's left hand allows the insertion of VS into oropharyngeal space. The hockey stick design of the VS makes insertion easy to access the epiglottis and approach glottic area. (D) Entry of the VS into trachea.

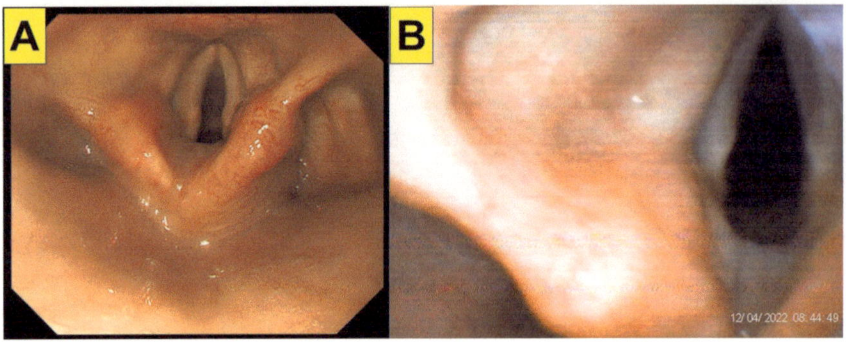

Figure 3.
Laryngeal and glottic views. (A) A perfect full-range glottic view from a flexible esophagogastroduodenoscopy examination in a 66-year-old man when the patient was under procedural analgesia. (B) A view from the video-assisted intubating stylet (VS) in an 89-year-old woman during tracheal intubation and general anesthesia. Laryngoscopic definition: POGO scale 100%; Cormack-Lehane class: I.

	AincA video stylet	**BESDATA reusable video stylet (BD-VSL)**	**IntuVu video stylet**	**Sensorendo® video stylet S-RVL**	**UE VL400-S3 video stylet**
Price	620 USD	700 USD	NA	NA	1800–5000 USD
Weight	NA	225 g	300 g	NA	180 g
Camera	NA	≥150 LUX, 1280 × 720 pixel	NA	1080 × 720 pixel resolution	NA
Display	2.4" full color video monitor	3" LCD, 640X480 (RGB)	3.5" IPS HD screen	3.5" video scree	2.5" LCD
Stylet	Malleable, waterproof	NA	NA	Waterproof	NA
Reusable	+	+	+	+	+
Clean and disinfection	Standard	NA	NA	Sterilizable	NA
ETT size	>6.0	NA	NA	4.5 mm diameter	3.0 mm, 5.2 mm

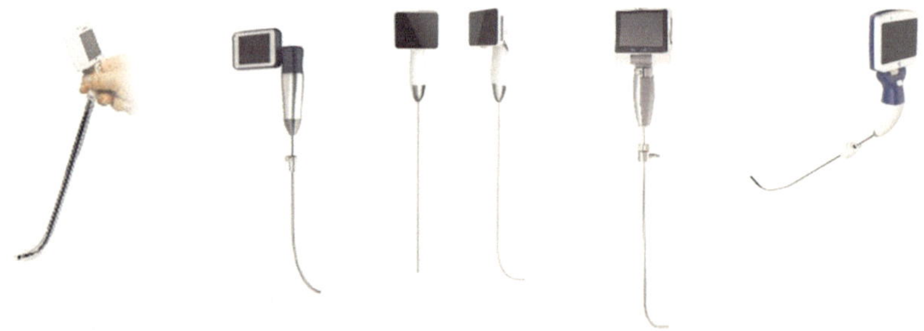

	ProVu™ Video Stylet	**Clarus Video System**	**Karl Storz C-MAC VS**	**TUORen Kingtaek Video Intubating System**	**HugeMed VL3H**
Price	600 USD	6000 USD	NA	5000 USD	800 USD
Weight	NA	NA	NA	NA	NA

Camera	NA	NA	NA	3840 × ≥150 LUX	640 × 480 (RGB), 2 M Piexel high resolution
Display	ProVu 3.5″ screen	4” LCD screen	NA	3.5″ screen	3.5″ screen
Stylet	NA	Waterproof	Completely watertight	Waterproof	NA
Reusable	+	+	+	+	+
Clean & Disinfection	NA	Soakable	Standard disinfection	Standard disinfection	NA
ETT size	6.5–8.0 mm	5.5–9.0 mm	Tube size 6.0 mm	NA	3.0–5.0 mm
	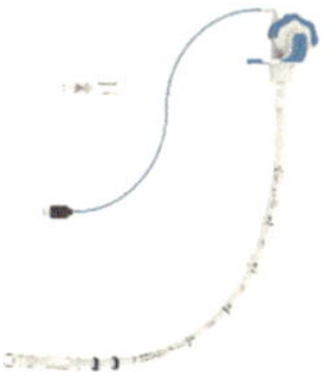	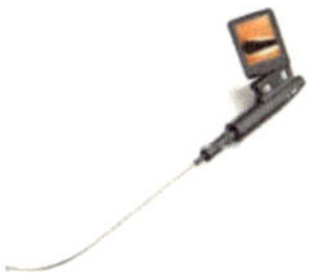	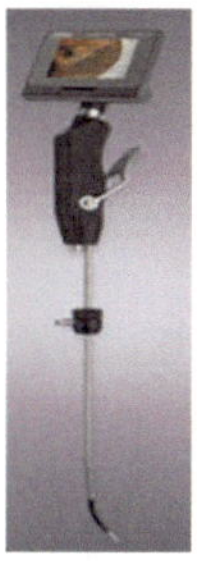	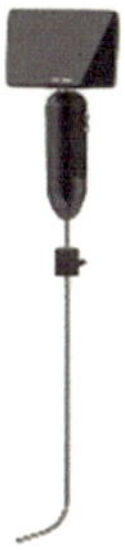	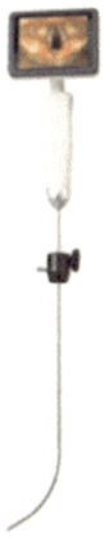

Table 1.
Examples of commercially available video-assisted intubating stylet.

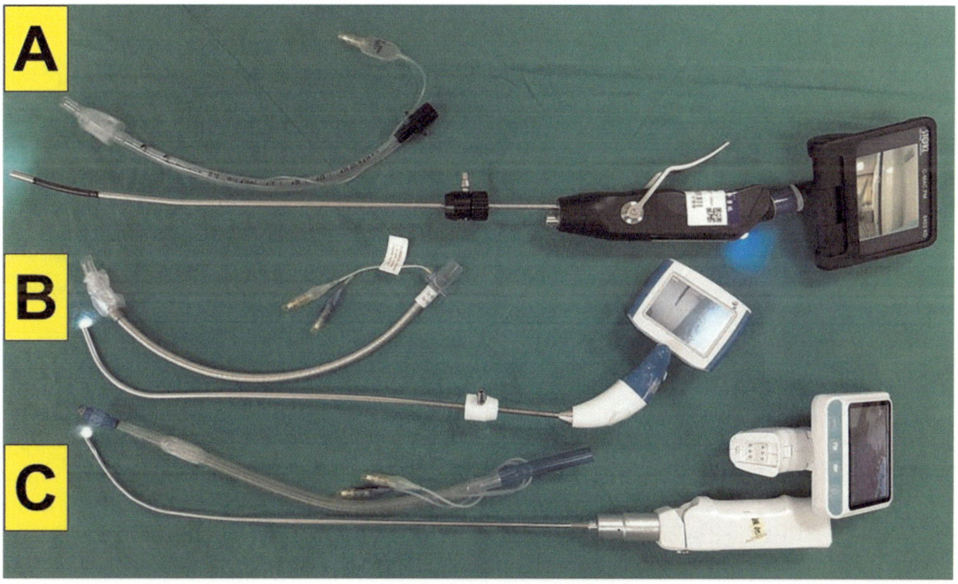

Figure 4.
Examples of commercial devices of VS. We apply the video-assisted intubating stylet technique at our institute on a daily routine basis. (A) C-MAC® VS, Karl Storz GmbH & Co. KG, Tuttlingen, Germany). (B) UE video stylet (UE, Xianju, Zhejiang, China). (C) Trachway video intubation system (Markstein Sichtec Medical Corp., Taichung, Taiwan). It is noted that these VS can accommodate various ET tubes, including regular ET tube (A), laser-resistant stainless steel ET tube (B), and double-lumen endobronchial tube (C).

	2016	2017	2018	2019	2020	2021
Total anesthesia number	16,077	17,831	17,998	19,307	19,721	19,244
GA number	15,339	16,893	17,497	18,481	19,009	18,574
LMA-GA number	5544	5134	5816	5902	5863	5714
ET-GA number	5953	6504	6920	6966	7418	6982
VL number	0	0	20	100	635	336
VS number	5953	6504	6900	6866	6783	6646

GA: general anesthesia. LMA: laryngeal mask anesthesia. ET: endotracheal intubation. VL: videolaryngoscope. VS: video-assisted intubating stylet.

Table 2.
Use coverage of video-assisted intubating stylet technique for tracheal intubation in the Department of Anesthesia, Hualien Tzuchi Medical Center, Hualien, Taiwan from 2016 to 2021.

used mostly for teaching purposes or personal preferences. With such a high volume of clinical practices using VS, we have acquired a significant experience with this technique and present it in the following sections.

2. Clinical experiences of optical intubating stylet

2.1 Airway grading

It is sometimes challenging to get a proper view of the glottis during routine tracheal intubation using DL. A simple prediction scale is therefore necessary and quite helpful in assessing and predicting risk during tracheal intubation [16–18]. We use the modified Cormack–Lehane (C–L) grading system of glottis view [19] to predict difficulty of tracheal intubation [20]. Modified scoring methods have also been used in our practice (e.g., percentage of glottis opening scale) [21, 22]. In addition to the competency in intubation technique, the quality of the airway assessment (e.g., difficult airway predictability) made by airway operators is also crucial for a successful intubation.

2.2 Preparation for placement of endotracheal tube

VS technique provides a superior view of the vocal cords and continuous visualization of the glottis for an easy and precise placement of the ET tube, as compared to DL and VL (**Figure 3B**). There are, however, some potential issues to be aware of when using VS: (1) Possible fogging of the lens (**Figure 5A**), which by the way can also happen with VL [23–26]. This is easy to prevent by careful wiping out the tip-lens with an anti-fog before use (**Figure 5B** and **C**). (2) Mucus or saliva covering the lens, and a good preventive maneuver is to keep the stylet a few millimeters proximal from the tip of ET tube, hence protecting the lens of the stylet. **Figure 5C** shows the appearance of the Murphy eye of an ET tube (side vent near the distal end of an ET tube) on a LCD screen. It should be emphasized that good video screen visualization is important for successful tracheal intubation when an optical stylet is used [27].

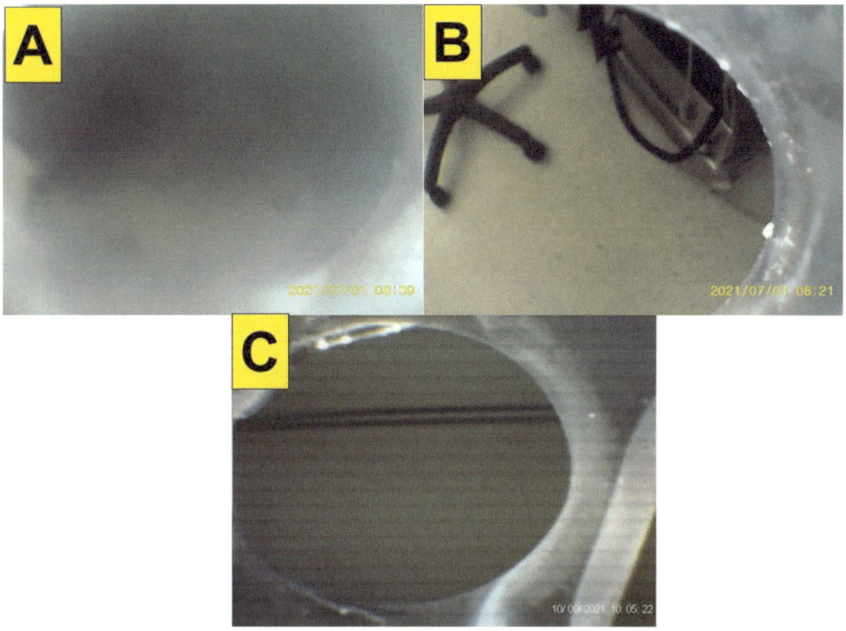

Figure 5.
The tip of VS should be kept clean and clear before use. (A) The optical lens was obscured and caused blurred vision. (B) Clear view after cleaning. (C) The relative position of the tips of the video stylet and endotracheal tube. The stylet tip was a little more backward than its position in (B).

2.3 Entrance to oral cavity

Since its original introduction in 1996 [6], numerous papers have been published on the application of the VS along with its advantages and benefits [13, 28–31]. An actual operating scenario for the Shikani technique of intubation is briefly described below. The operator first lifts up patient's mandible with the left hand and displaces it anteriorly until the lower teeth are anterior to the upper teeth (**Figure 6A**). The stylet-loaded ET tube set is then advanced forward by the right hand until the epiglottis is seen on the monitor. The operator can then maneuver the stylet beneath and pass around the epiglottis while continuously visualizing the airway. This allows a smooth and atraumatic railroading of the ET tube through the glottis and into the trachea. Occasionally, the tongue is large and in the way and the glottis cannot be seen clearly. In these situations, combining a Macintosh blade would further open the upper airway and bring the glottis into view. Alternatively, in contrast to the single-handed chin lift maneuver, a two-handed jaw thrust aided by an assistant can be used to facilitate the VS intubation (**Figure 6B**). With this strategy, the assistant stands either side by side or opposite the operator [32, 33]. It should be cautioned that the BURP (backward, upward, rightward external laryngeal pressure) is not helpful or recommended for VS technique. The combined use of VL or DL was also reported using the Bonfils rigid endoscope [34] or a lighted stylet [35]. **Figure 6C** shows the combination of DL and VS. Detailed description of such combination method will be presented in the latter part of this article.

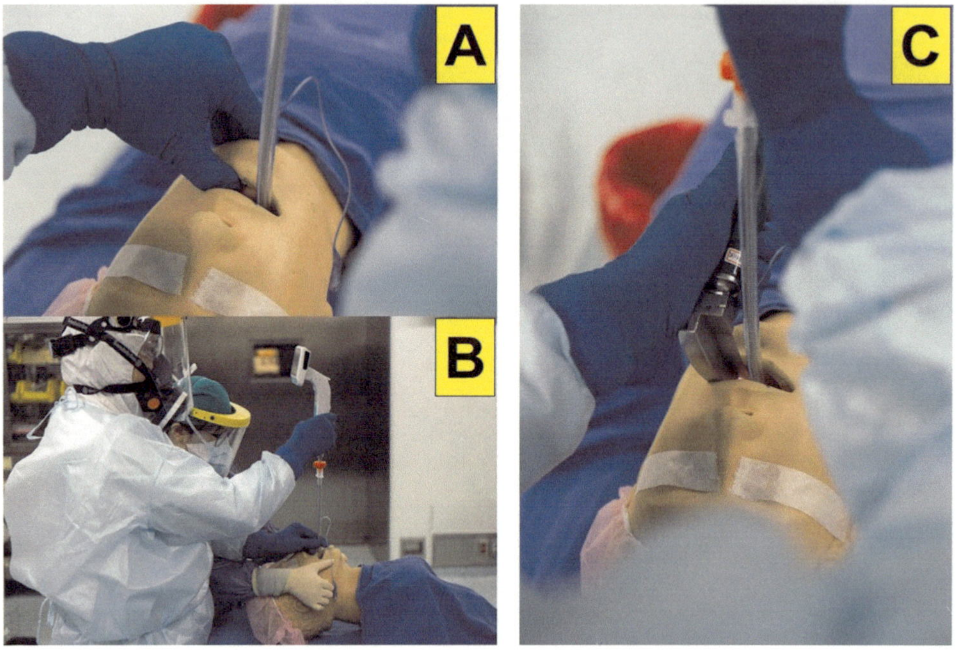

Figure 6.
Three methods to perform the VS technique. (A) Classical Shikani method. (B) Two-person performance. An assistant stood side by side with the operator (or opposite the operator) to provide jaw-thrust maneuver. (C) Combined use of laryngoscopy and VS technique. All three maneuvers can open patient's airway and enlarge retropharyngeal space for further advancement of the video stylet.

2.4 Glottic view

While the original and modified Cormack-Lehane grading system are useful [36], they are clinically meaningful and transferrable only if optimal intubating technique (e.g., optimal blade and its position, lifting force, head/neck position, external laryngeal manipulation, awake or anesthetized) is employed [37]. The main purpose of the C-L grading system is to describe the glottic view during direct laryngoscopy and might not necessarily translate to ease and speed of tracheal intubation. When VL was introduced [38], some reported that it had higher rates of successful intubation on the first attempt with improved glottic views, as compared to DL [7]. However, in different clinical settings (e.g., in emergency room or intensive care unit) and different patient populations (e.g., pediatric patients), VL did not show its superiority in first-pass success rate and time to intubation, as compared to DL [39].

In contrast to DL and VL, VS seems to provide the best glottic view as the tip of the stylet can access the laryngeal inlet and be positioned beneath the epiglottis. Because the vocal cords are directly visualized, the passage of the stylet-ET tube into trachea is almost assured. This allows minimal (if any) trauma while circumventing any laryngeal pathology such as cysts, tumors, etc.

We believe the glottis visualization grading systems for VS technique should be simply graded as "easy, restricted, and difficult". The crux of the matter in airway intubation is "to see is to accomplish". If the vocal cords can be seen, the placement of ET tube is then easy. We propose such a grading system (LQS system) specific for VS technique shown in **Figure 7**.

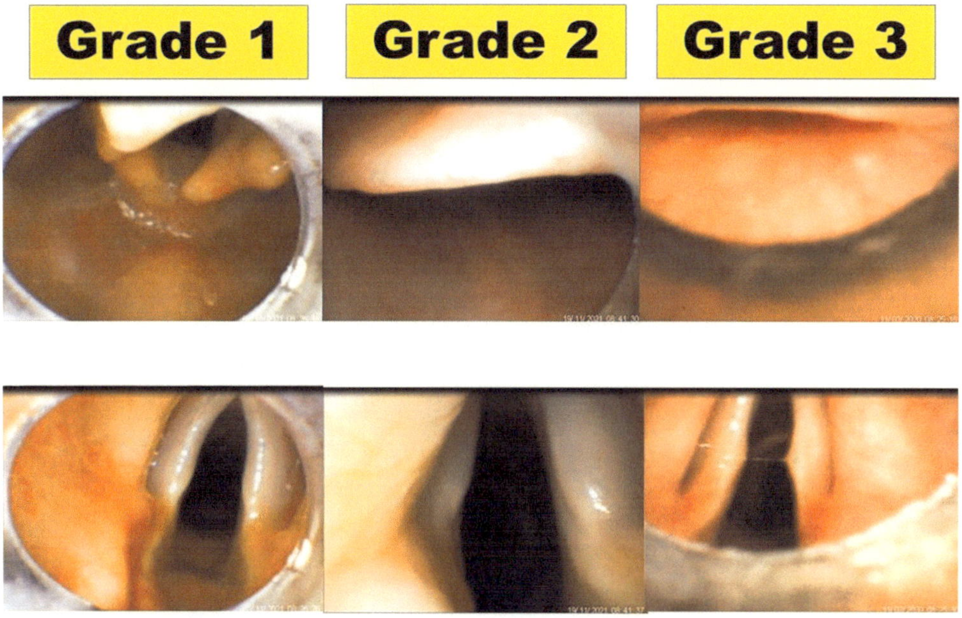

Figure 7.
LQS grading score on glottis visualization by VS technique. Grade 1: Able to see any part of the vocal cords and arytenoid cartilages. Grade 2: None of glottis parts can be seen. Only epiglottis can be seen and there is enough space left between the epiglottis and posterior pharyngeal wall. Grade 3: The space under the epiglottis is very narrow and probably will create difficulty passing the stylet. It should be emphasized that once the stylet can be introduced beneath the epiglottis, full glottis view can be obtained (images shown in the lower row). This is a case for double-lumen endobronchial tube placement. Intubation time (for demonstration purposes): 28, 26, and 30 s, respectively. Please also compare with ***Figure 8****. (Also see the Supplementary Materials Videos S1–S3. To watch the supplementary videos contact the email address: lukairforce@gmail.com).*

- **Grade 1**: Any part of the glottis (vocal cords and arytenoid cartilages) can easily be seen. The stylet-ET tube set can easily be passed into the trachea.

- **Grade 2**: The glottis cannot be visualized, but there is enough space between the floppy epiglottis and posterior pharyngeal wall. This allows the stylet-ET tube combination to be maneuvered to pass around the epiglottis and enter the trachea.

- **Grade 3**: The space between the epiglottis and glottis opening is extremely small, requiring a significant jaw-thrust or combining VS with a Macintosh blade to open the airway and allow visualization of the glottis.

The majority of the cases (74%) fell into grade 1 (**Figure** 7, left panel), 25% into grade 2 (**Figure** 7, middle panel), and very few (1%) classified into grade 3 (**Figure** 7, right panel) that required more laborious maneuverability to pass the stylet-ET tube set through the glottis. Our proposed grading method (LQS grading score), similar to other systems (e.g., C–L score, POGO score), does not require exact knowledge of grading minutiae (e.g., subdivided into 2a, 2b, 3a, 3b) [36, 40]. Our clinical experiences of the use of VS for routine and emergency intubation indicated that the LQS grading system was correlated with various intubating outcomes, such as intubating time, first-attempt success rate, easiness, complication rates, etc.

In our experience using the VS technique, we encountered some problems that caused the intubation to be more difficult, including: (1) copious mucus and saliva obscuring the lens and views; (2) stiff neck and restricted cervical mobility limiting the jaw-thrust; and (3) swollen soft tissues and floppy epiglottis hindering the pass of the stylet-ET tube either from midline or from the side of epiglottis (**Figure 8B**, left panel). In those difficult cases, the FOB technique may be helpful (**Figure 8B**, middle and right panels).

It should be emphasized that the LQS grading system is for VS technique combined with the simple jaw-thrust maneuver and may be affected by various patient conditions (e.g., restricted head/neck motility, pathological obstruction of airway, efficiency of jaw-thrust maneuver). Therefore, in patients with simulated difficult airway (e.g., using cervical collar or manual in-line stabilization) and a confirmed a high C–L grade by DL, the subsequent use of VS may take a longer time [41]. However, similar high intubation success rates with VS technique were obtained in both low C–L grade and high C–L grade patients in the simulated difficult airway scenario. During such intubation with VS, visualization of vocal cords and advancement into the glottis for the high-grade group was significantly more difficult than in the low-grade group [41].

In patients with a large and floppy epiglottis (i.e., LQS grade 3), the view can be improved by simply applying a jaw-thrust maneuver or by combining with a Macintosh blade [42, 43]. **Figure 9** shows such an example using a jaw-thrust maneuver to lift up the epiglottis for passage of the stylet-ET tube set. In this case, the

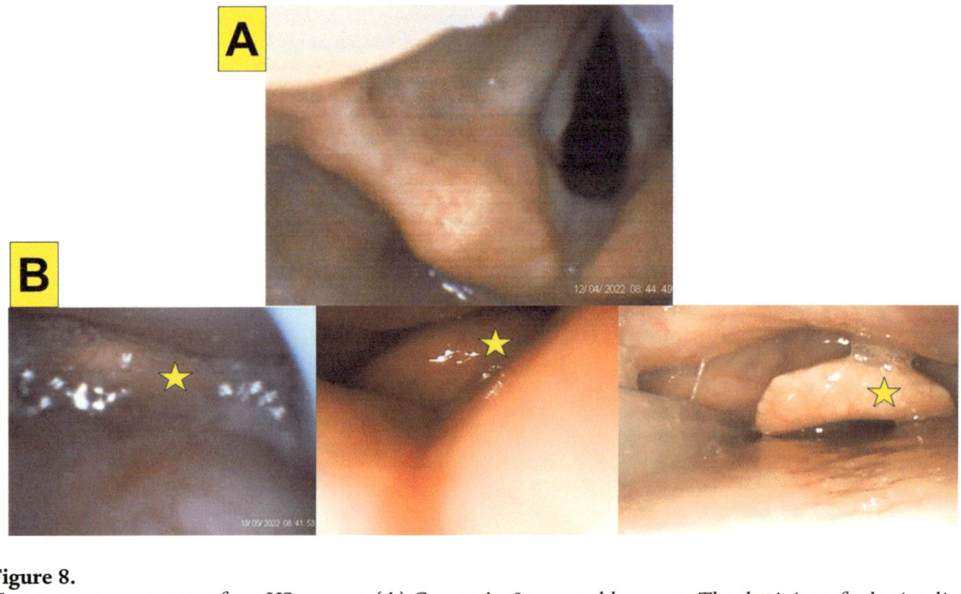

Figure 8.
Two uncommon cases seen from VS camera. (A) Case 1: An 89-year-old woman. The glottis is perfectly visualized simply by jaw-thrust maneuver and the vocal cords fully open and visible (i.e., Cormack-Lehane class 1, POGO 100%). (B) Case 2: A 75-year-old man. The epiglottis could not be lifted up at all by jaw-thrust maneuver due to severe radiation fibrosis of the neck. The epiglottis is labeled by the yellow star. Left panel: The epiglottis was completely attached to the posterior pharyngeal wall when the patient was anesthetized and paralyzed. Intubation with VS technique failed after several attempts. Middle panel: The patient was quickly reversed from anesthetized status to asleep status with spontaneous respiration. Rescue intubation was eventually achieved by FOB. The epiglottis still remained drooped. Right panel: Three weeks later, the same patient received elective tracheostomy due to difficulty breathing. Awake nasal intubation was done with FOB. The patient in ***Figure 8B*** *is the same as in* ***Figures 36–40****.*

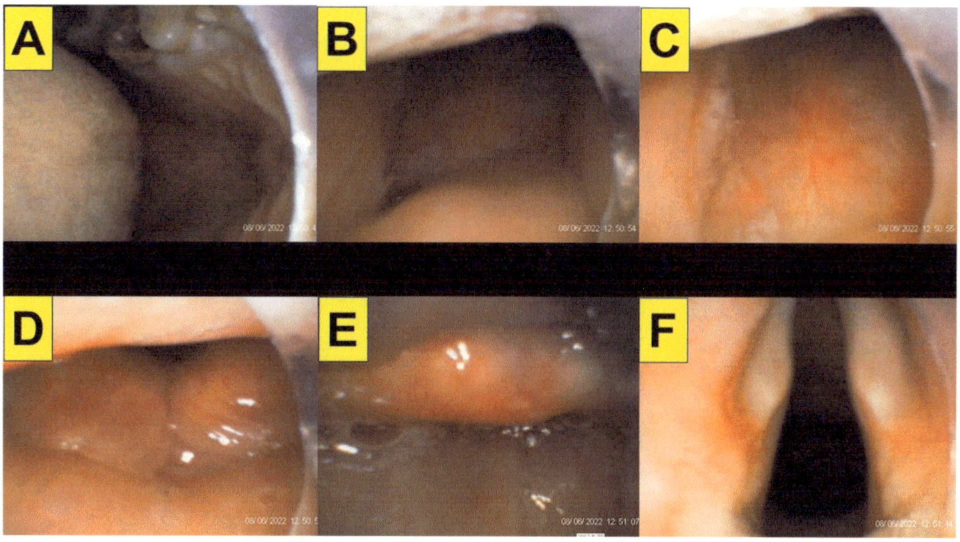

Figure 9.
Effect of jaw-thrust maneuver on improving glottis view seem from VS. this is a 66-year-old man with a BMI 25.0 kg/m^2 (167 cm, 70 kg). Mallampati score: Class 2. Neck circumference 44 cm. (A) View of oral cavity by opening mouth. (B) View of pharynx entry and uvula. (C) Laryngeal inlet. (D) Jaw-thrust created a LQS score grade 1 with partial view of glottic region. (E) Without jaw-thrust maneuver, epiglottis stayed back and attached to posterior pharyngeal wall. (F) Close-up panorama view of glottis. Intubation time (from lip to trachea, for demonstration): 30 s (Supplementary Materials Video S4).

oro-pharyngeal-laryngeal space/inlet was open and accessible (**Figure 9A–C**). However, jaw-thrust could only lift up the epiglottis to expose the vocal cords less than 50% (**Figure 9D** and **E**) in this patient. Once the space underneath the epiglottis was wide enough to allow VS passage, the vocal cords could easily be viewed fully (**Figure 9F**). Further placement of the ET tube was easy by railroading the tube from VS.

2.5 Time to intubation

A mounting body of evidence indicates that VL reduces the rate of failed intubation and results in higher rates of successful intubation on the first attempt with an improved glottic view [7]. In patients with anticipated difficult airways (e.g., cervical collar limited mouth opening and neck movement), VL was safe and quicker in controlling the airway (time to view the vocal cords: 20–30 s (median); time to advance tube 30–40 s (median); intubation time of successful attempt: 50–60 s) [44]. The reported intubation time for emergency intubation by VL is 60 s $\pm$ 31 s (difficulty score with Visual Analogue Scale 0–100: 39 $\pm$ 27) [45]. In adult patients with a normal airway, the time for successful tracheal intubation with VL is short (17–38 s) [46]. Similar time ranges were found for emergency intubation with VL in these patients (12–15 s) [47].

Figure 10 shows four examples of the use of VS technique in patients with normal airways under routine tracheal intubation for elective surgeries. In two patients who needed rapid sequence intubation, the intubation time (from lip to trachea) using VS was 5–7 s, respectively (**Figure 10**, the left two panels). For teaching purposes or if there is a need to "look around the corner", the intubation time was slowed down to 20–30 s (**Figure 10**, the right two panels). If the intubation takes a longer time

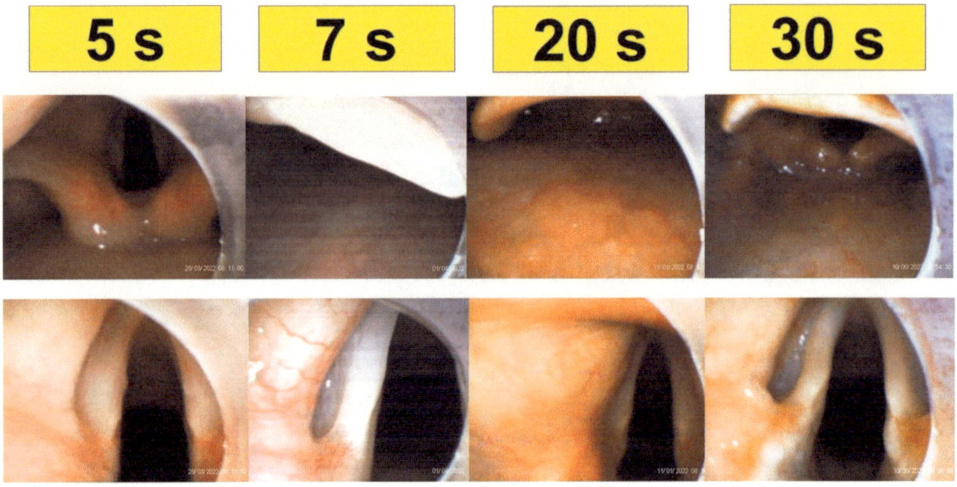

Figure 10.
Time to intubation (from lip to trachea) using VS technique in four examples. Upper row: View from epiglottis. Lower row: Close-up view of glottis. Left (5 s): A 36-year-old man with BMI 22.7 kg/m² (178 cm, 72 kg). Second from the left (7 s): A 52-year-old woman with BMI 24.0 kg/m² (162 cm, 63 kg). Third from the left (20 s): A 42-year-old man with BMI 29.3 kg/m² (174 cm, 89 kg). Right (30 s): A 55-year-old man with BMI 23.0 kg/m² (164 cm, 62 kg). It is noted that the speed of intubation was deliberately slowed down (20 and 30 s) for demonstration purpose. (Also see the Supplementary Materials Videos S5–S8).

(e.g., between 30 and 60 s), the operator should anticipate a potentially difficult intubation (e.g., **Figure 8B**) and a plan B should always be prepared.

During airway management, the airway is not always as clear as seen in **Figure 10**. In the real world, the airway operator using VS technique might encounter copious thick mucus, saliva, or sometimes blood in the airway. Those secretions may obscure the lens of the optical intubating tool and make intubation more difficult. Frank emesis and massive vomitus or blood can occur in certain traumatic emergencies [48, 49]. Quick, effective, and continuous suctioning of pharyngeal secretions or blood is necessary to reduce the risk of losing visualization. A tracheal suction catheter or Yankauer suction tip would help clearing the oropharynx and larynx. **Figure 11** shows the saliva impeding the glottic view when VS technique was applied. Pre-medication with an anti-sialagogue and proper suctioning are helpful to reduce such problems before inserting the optical stylet into the patient's oropharynx.

3. Routine use of VS in elective and emergency surgeries

VL and DL have been used for decades in both elective and emergency intubations. The introduction of VL has shifted the paradigm of airway management [50]. VS was first introduced by Shikani in patients (both adults and children) undergoing routine otolaryngologic procedures [6] and has since been applied in various clinical scenarios, including difficult and emergency airway [12, 51]. The VS technique has been studied in adults in supine position [52–56], in lateral decubitus position [57], and in pediatric patients with difficult airway [30, 58]. It has also been used during awake intubation [53, 59] and for diagnostic bronchoscopy [60]. VS has also been used by emergency room physicians [61] and emergency medical technicians in the pre-hospital airway management [62].

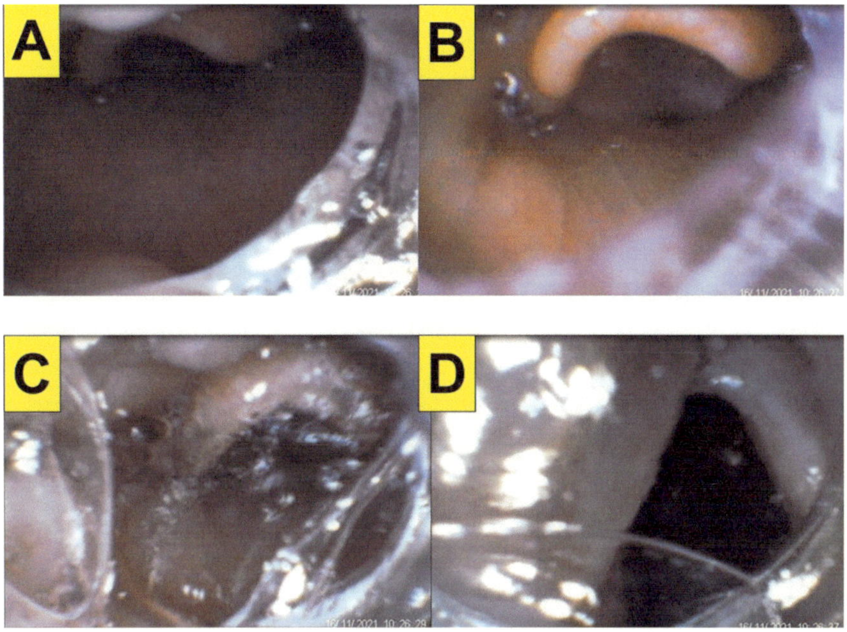

Figure 11.
Presence of mucus and saliva interfering with laryngeal views obtained by VS technique during tracheal intubation. A morbidly obese 42-year-old woman with BMI 46.6 kg/m² (165 cm, 127 kg) underwent fasciotomy and debridement. Past history included sleep apnea and snoring. LQS score grade 1. The intubation time (for demonstration) is 22 s. (Also see the Supplementary Materials Video S9).

In 2010, VS was introduced into our department. At that time, most of our staff still used DL and some tried VL (e.g., GlideScope®) [63, 64]. We established a formal airway training course in DL, VL, and VS use for the staff and novice operators using cadaver and mannequins. Currently, we have more than 22 sets of VS from four different brands in our 21 operating rooms. Although it is not mandated to use VS, VS prevails among all the available intubating tools we have. We regularly survey the novice users and trainees to evaluate their performance and obtain feedback. Notably, VS is used in more than 90% of tracheal intubations (**Table 2**).

Figure 12 demonstrates the routine use of VS for tracheal intubation in an elective surgery. We have previously reported on the application of VS in patients undergoing an emergency surgery during the COVID-19 pandemic [65–70] (see **Figures 13** and **14**). The coverall personal protective equipment (PPE) and plastic sheet barrier did not interfere with smooth tracheal intubation using VS in COVID-19 patients. In both clinical scenarios (**Figures 12–14**), VS technique provides a swift, and safe tracheal intubation, while protecting the intubating provider from secretions as he/she does not have to put his/her face close to the patient's mouth.

Table 3 summarizes the strengths and weakness of VL and VS. The clinical performance of VS is usually evaluated in many aspects, including (1) insertion in the oropharynx; (2) visualization of the epiglottis; (3) advancement in the glottic aperture; (4) maneuverability of the stylet; and (5) adverse events such as dental trauma, soft tissues damages, autonomic overstimulation, aspiration, hypoxia, etc. In both normal airway and difficult airway scenarios, VS shows its advantages with shorter intubating time [13, 71–74], less autonomic stimulation [55], and shorter learning curve [75].

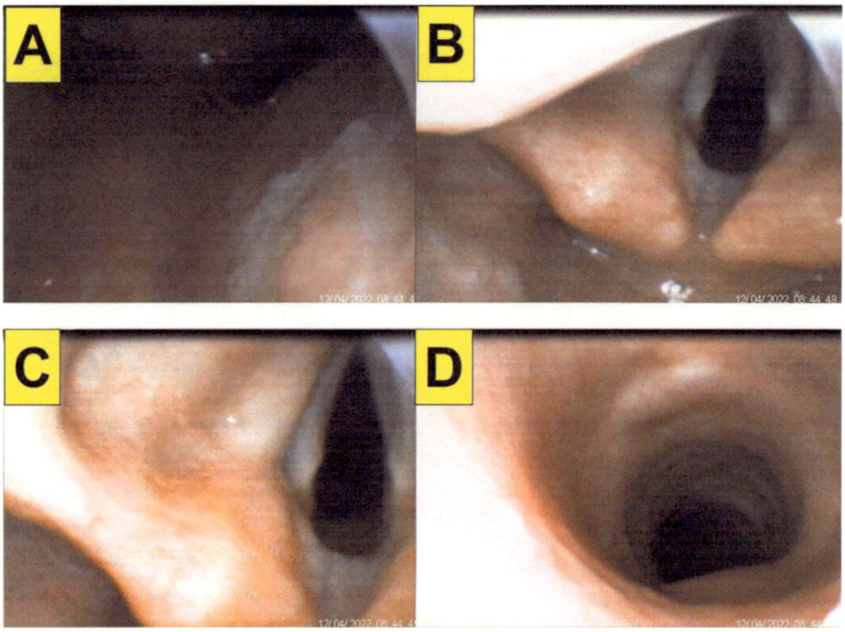

Figure 12.
A typical case of routinely applying VS technique for tracheal intubation in elective surgery. An 89-year-old woman with BMI 25.3 kg/m² (150 cm, 57 kg). The intubation time (from lip to trachea) is 7 s. (Also see the Supplementary Materials Video S10).

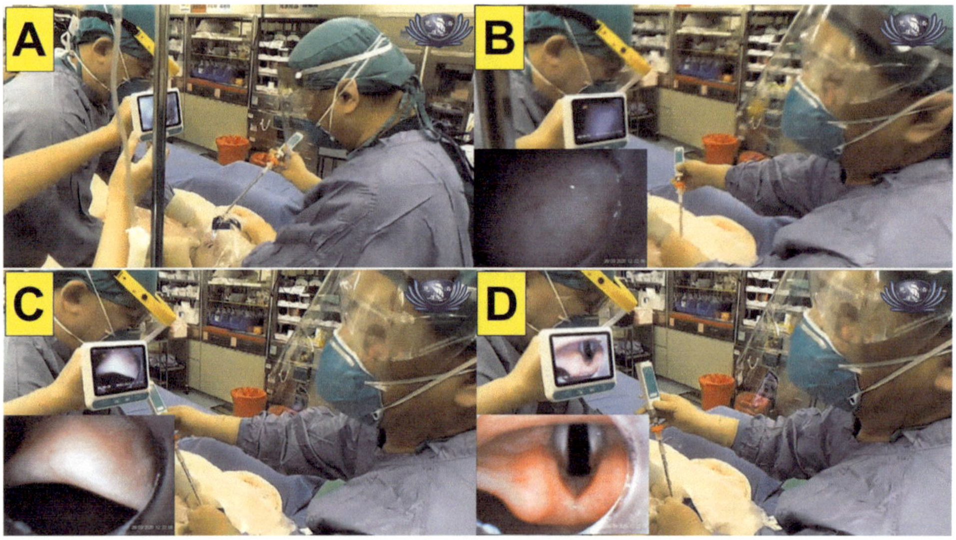

Figure 13.
A typical case of routinely applying VS for tracheal intubation during emergency surgery. A 26-year-old woman with BMI 21.3 kg/m² (150 cm, 48 kg) underwent an emergent orthopedic surgery due to multiple trauma during COVID-19 pandemic in 2020. Combined use of VS and a piece of plastic sheet as a protective barrier was noted. The two anesthesiologists wore PPE during tracheal intubation procedure. The anesthesia assistant was performing jaw-thrust maneuver. (Also see the Supplementary Materials Video S11).

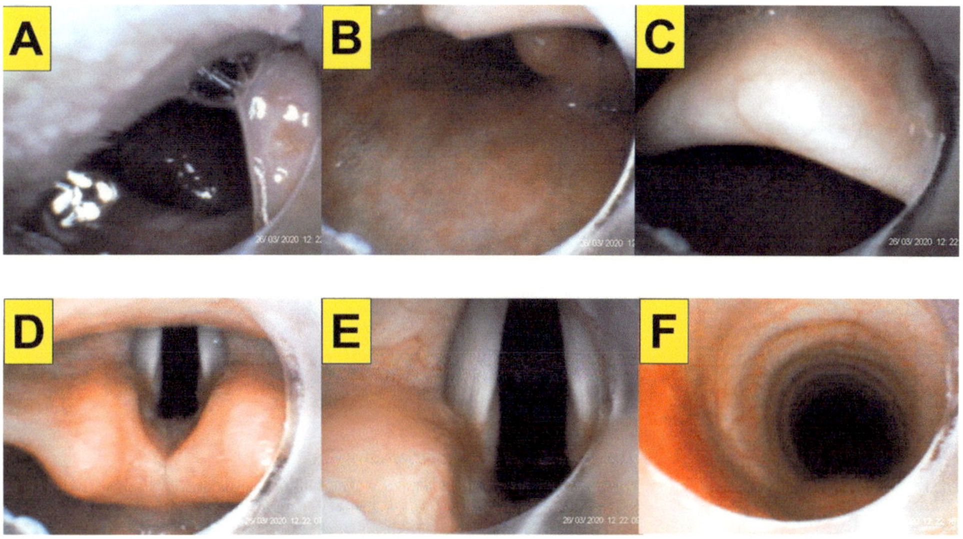

Figure 14.
Same patient as in ***Figure 13****. Close-up views from the VS video LCD screen. (A and B) Views of oropharynx and larynx. (C) Epiglottis. (D and E) Views of glottis and vocal cords. (F) Entry into trachea. The intubation time was 12 s. (Also see the Supplementary Materials Video S12).*

	VL	VS
Required use of a blade	+	–
Forces to laryngoscopy	++	–
Require mouth-opening	+++	+
Forces applied to the maxillary incisors	++	–
Use of a stylet	±	–
Maneuverability during navigation	+	+++
Ability to control the tip and displace soft tissues	+	+++
Require lift-up epiglottis	+++	+
Better Cormack-Lehane/LQS grading	+	+++
Difficult placement/insertion	+++	–
Ability to visualize the insertion of the tip of ET tube into trachea	+	+++
High first-attempt success rate	++	+++
More number of attempts	++	+
High overall success rate	++	+++
Short time to intubation	++	+++
Need of external laryngeal maneuver	++	–
Esophageal intubation	++	–
Autonomic stimulation	++	–
Airway trauma/injury	++	–

	VL	VS
Other complications	++	–
Affordable (cost)	+	++
Short setup time and portability	+++	+++
Availability, accessible, maintenance	++	++
Skill/technique learning curve	++	+++

VL: Videolaryngoscope. VS: Video-assisted intubating stylet. Complications: Hypoxemia, hypotension. "+" and "–" denote the degree of relative comparison between use of VL and VS.

Table 3.
Comparison between videolaryngoscopes (VL) and video-assisted intubating stylet (VS).

4. First-line choice of VS in difficult airway

Over the last decade, the VS technique has been widely used as an alternative to VL in simulated difficult airways (e.g., rigid cervical collars applied) [6, 31, 76–83], cervical spine surgeries [84, 85], upper airway obstruction [86–89], double-lumen endobronchial tube placement [90–92], and emergent awake intubation [93]. In the following sections, we present our clinical experiences of using the VS technique as the first-line intubating modality in several difficult airway scenarios.

4.1 Head neck lesions

Various video-assisted intubating stylets have been used in potential or anticipated difficult airway as the first-line tool for tracheal intubation. We previously reported use of VS in patients with anticipated difficult airway, such as facial-oral tumors, enlarged tonsils, radiation neck fibrosis, hypopharyngeal cancers, and laryngeal tumors and cysts [94]. Similarly, VS was also reported in patients with an epiglottic cyst [86, 87], retropharyngeal tumor [88], and in awake nasal intubation [89].

Although awake/asleep flexible fiberoptic bronchoscopy and elective/emergency tracheostomy still remain the gold standard of the airway management in extreme difficult airway (e.g., hypopharyngeal cancer, severe radiation-induced fibrosis over neck, giant neck tumors, restricted mouth opening), VS can play a role in anticipated difficult airway, similar to the proposed role of awake FOB and VL [95]. One advantage of the Shikani stylet over the fiberoptic scope is the ability to maneuver it around a floppy epiglottis, especially if the patient is asleep and in the supine position. It should be mentioned that rigid endoscopy is one of the difficult airway rescue modalities [96].

Figure 15 shows an example of a potential difficult airway in a patient with hypopharyngeal cancer undergoing laryngo-microsurgery (LMS) intubated with VS. The epiglottis was difficult to lift up but the space between the epiglottis and posterior pharyngeal wall was just wide enough to allow the stylet-ET tube set to go through. A good glottis view was obtained, and intubation was completed without delay. When VS is used in patients with head/neck lesions, the operator should expect that mucus and blood can blur the lens of VS and be prepared to handle that (**Figure 16**).

When a patient has been previously treated with radiotherapy or surgery, a stiff neck caused by radiation fibrosis, flap, or scar is expected. In **Figure 17**, the patient's mouth opening was wide enough, but the neck was stiff and the cervical spine

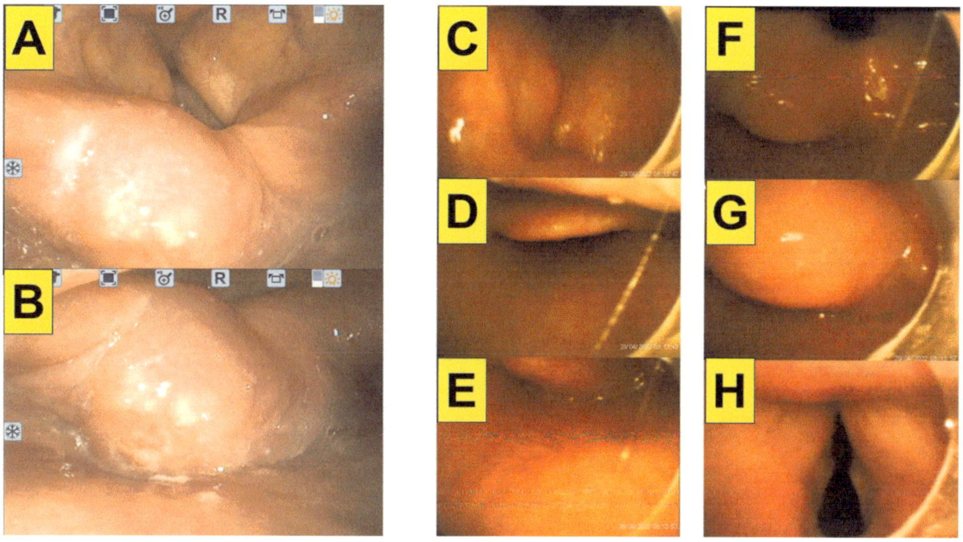

Figure 15.
Use of VS technique in a patient with anticipated difficult airway. A 66-year-old man (BMI 22.6 kg/m²; 164 cm, 61 kg) with hypopharyngeal cancer underwent LMS surgery. (A) and (B) Pre-operative endoscopic survey images. (C–H): Serial views during tracheal intubation using VS under general anesthesia. The epiglottis could not be fully lifted up by sole jaw-thrust maneuver (D). The intubation time: 20 s. (also see the Supplementary Materials Video S13).

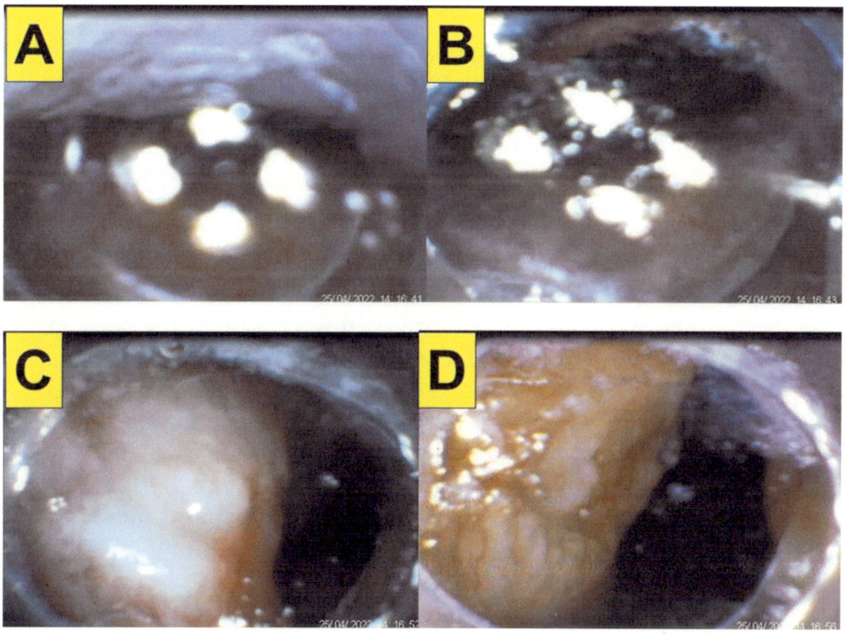

Figure 16.
Use of VS technique complicated by a saliva bubble in a patient with hypopharyngeal cancer. This is a 57-year-old man with BMI 26.0 kg/m² (172 cm, 77 kg). The intubation time: 20 s. (Also see the Supplementary Materials Video S14).

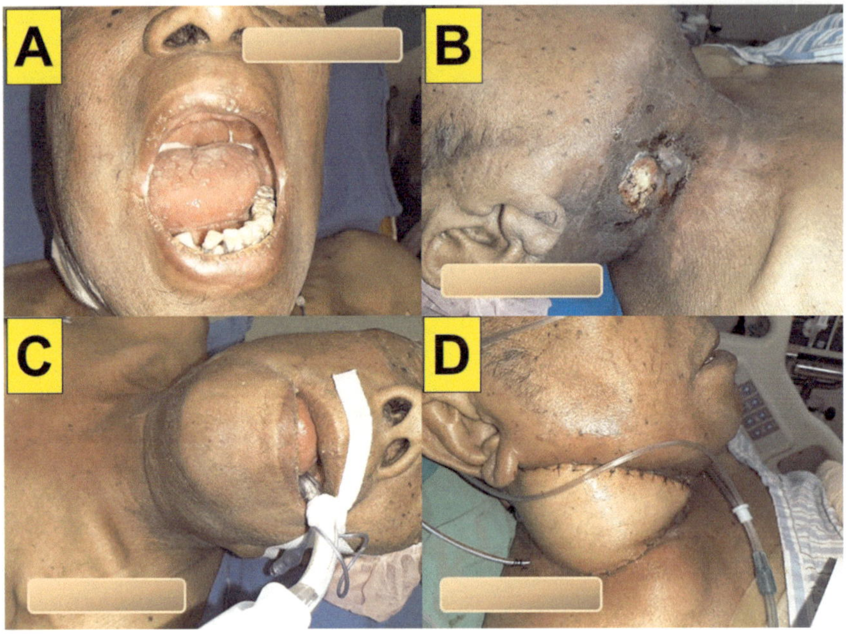

Figure 17.
Use of VS technique in a patient with stiff neck caused by radiation therapy. This is a 72-year-old man with BMI 20.4 kg/m^2 *(174 cm, 62 kg). He had squamous cell carcinoma over the neck with metastasis and received definitive concurrent chemoradiotherapy. (A) Mouth opening is wide enough. (B) Stiff neck due to radiation fibrosis with ulceration. (C) Post-intubation. (D) Post-operation after extubation.*

mobility was restricted. His glottic inlet was narrow due to edema of the pharyngeal tissues and epiglottis. The intubation was nevertheless smoothly executed using VS technique (**Figure 18**).

4.2 Morbid obesity

Obesity and morbid obesity can complicate airway management. Impaired glottis visualization [97–102] leads to greater lifting force and external laryngeal pressure. Several prediction algorithms have been proposed for the morbidly obese patient [103–105], including anthropometric parameters [106–109]. Body mass index and neck circumference are commonly used to predict difficult airways [110–113], although some studies showed no association with difficult intubation [114]. Still, it is a general consensus that morbid obesity makes tracheal intubation difficult [109]. There are various intubating modalities for obese patients [115–120] and VL is superior to conventional DL [121–130]. VS is useful in morbid patients due to its improved visualization of the larynx and the ease with tube advancement [131, 132].

Our clinical experiences support the role of VS in morbidly obese patients. **Figure 19** shows tracheal intubation with VS in a patient whose oropharynx was too narrow for laryngoscopy (**Figure 19F**). In the last six years, we have performed hundreds of intubations on morbidly obese patients (including more than 100 patients undergoing bariatric surgery), and there were only two cases that we were not able to intubate with VS. **Figure 20** shows three examples of the application of VS in morbidly obese patients (BMI 36.6, 49.9, and 58.4 kg/m^2, respectively). The

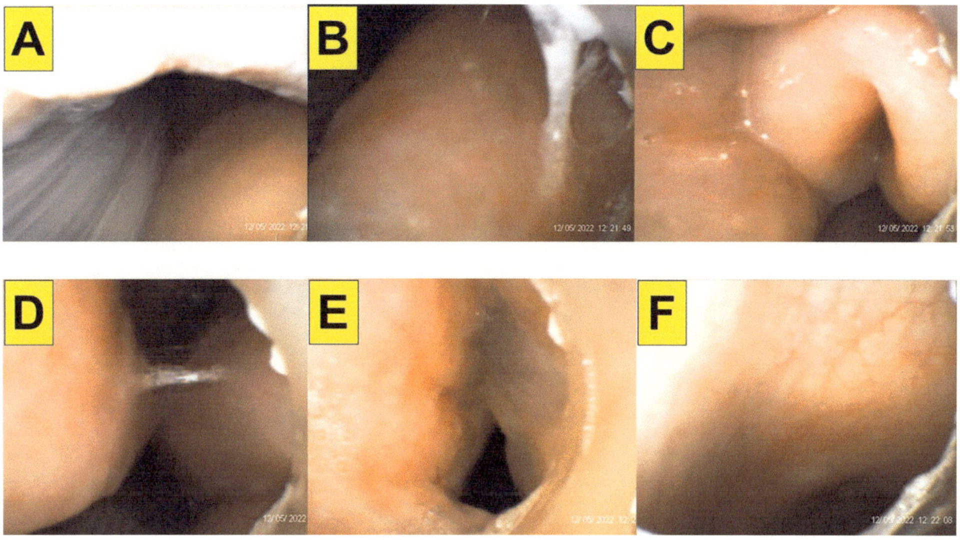

Figure 18.
Close-up views from VS in the same patient from ***Figure 17****. Due to limited effects of jaw-thrust maneuver in the presence of radiation fibrosis of the neck, the oro-pharynx (A and B), larynx (C and D) are crowded. The epiglottis curls inward and manifests omega-shaped folding (C). (E) The glottis opening is narrow. (F) ET tube is secured into trachea. The intubation time is 24 s. (Also see the Supplementary Materials Video S15).*

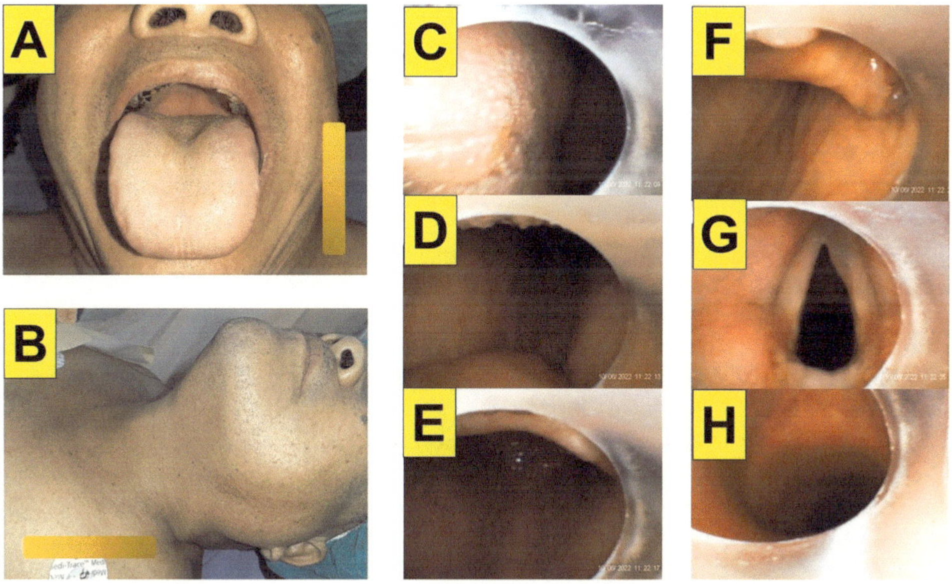

Figure 19.
A 65-year-old morbidly obese man with BMI 40.5 kg/m² (167 cm, 113 kg). (A) Modified Mallampati test: Class 3. Mouth opening 5.5 cm. (B) Thyromental distance: 6.5 cm. Sternomental distance: 11.5 cm. Neck circumference: 47 cm. Upper lip bite test: Class 1. (C–H) Serial views from VS camera. (C) View of oropharynx. (D, E) laryngeal inlet is crowded with LQS score grade 1. (F) Without jaw-thrust maneuver, the LQS class is grade 2. (G, H) Clear visualization of glottis and tracheal rings. The intubation time (for demonstration) is 30 s. (Also see the Supplementary Materials Video S16).

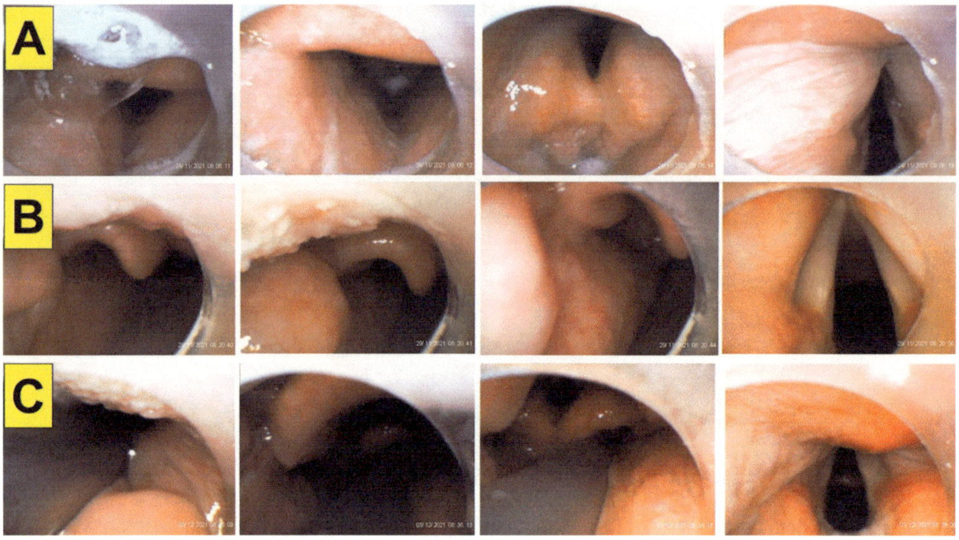

Figure 20.
Serial close-up views from VS in three typical morbidly obese patients. (A) BMI 36.6 kg/m² (170 cm, 106 kg). A 37-year-old man underwent laparoscopic hernioplasty. The intubation time is 20 s. (B) BMI 49.9 kg/m² (165 cm, 136 kg). A 37-year-old woman underwent laparoscopic sleeve gastrectomy. The intubation time is 20 s. (C) BMI 58.4 kg/m² (167 cm, 163 kg). The intubation time is 22 s. It is interesting to note that the LQS grading scores in all these three morbid obesity cases are grade 1. It is noted that laryngeal tissues are crowded. (Also see the Supplementary Materials Video S17–S19).

intubation with VS technique was smooth and fast. The "video-video paired technique" will be presented in the latter part of this article.

4.3 Restricted cervical spine mobility

Restricted cervical spine (C-spine) mobility is a major risk factor for difficult airway in various prediction algorithms. Although awake/asleep/anesthetized flexible fiberoptic bronchoscopy is the gold standard for airway management, other airway modalities and tools have been proposed in the literature [133]. Among all the airway tools, VL has drawn the most attention as a useful tool for restricted C-spine motion. This technique has been tested in patients with a simulated restricted C-spine condition (with manual in-line stabilization or rigid cervical collar) [44, 134–145], in real patients undergoing C-spine surgeries [146, 147], and in mannequin simulation model [148, 149]. Recently, VS has also been tested in patients with simulated restricted C-spine motion [31, 78, 80, 81, 84, 150, 151].

Our single-institute clinical experience (more than 600 C-spine surgeries a year) indicates that the VS technique is a very useful technique in this patient population. **Figure 21** shows a case when cervical spine mobility was restricted by the neck collar. Another example of limited C-spine mobility is in patients receiving stereotactic neurosurgeries with a head frame mounted before tracheal intubation can occur. **Figure 22** shows such a scenario.

4.4 COVID-19 pandemic

The COVID-19 pandemic created a major challenge in airway management for both patients and providers [152]. It was reported that VL "should be dedicated for

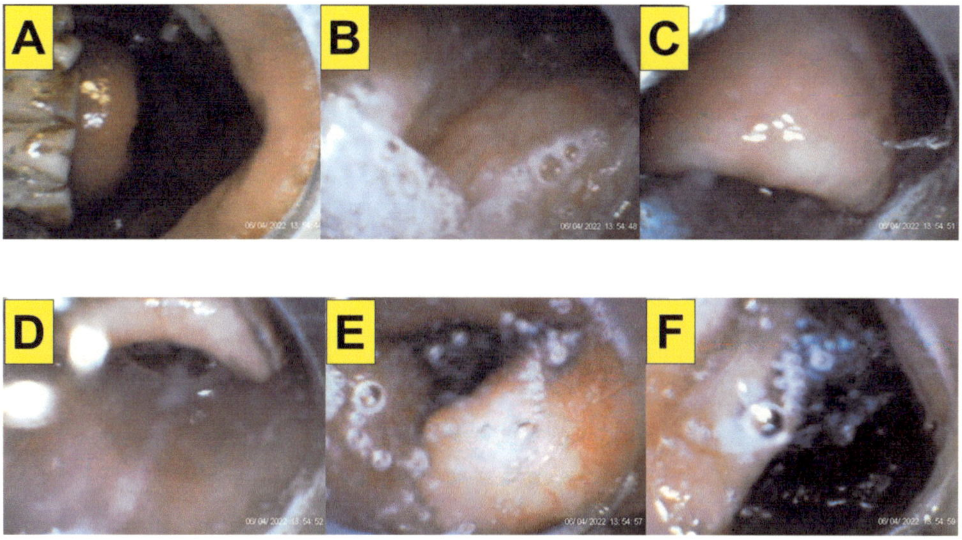

Figure 21.
Application of VS technique in a 42-year-old male patient (BMI 29.6 kg/m²) with cervical collar immobilization due to C4-5 contusion. (A) Fair mouth opening. (B) Copious saliva and secretions in the pharynx and larynx. (C, D) The immobilization process itself caused a worse glottic view (LQS scale: 2. No glottis structures can be seen at all). Fortunately, the space underneath the epiglottis is enough for passage of the stylet-ET tube. (E, F) The secretion bubbles disturbed the glottis view. The intubation time is 16 s. (Also see the Supplementary Materials Video S20).

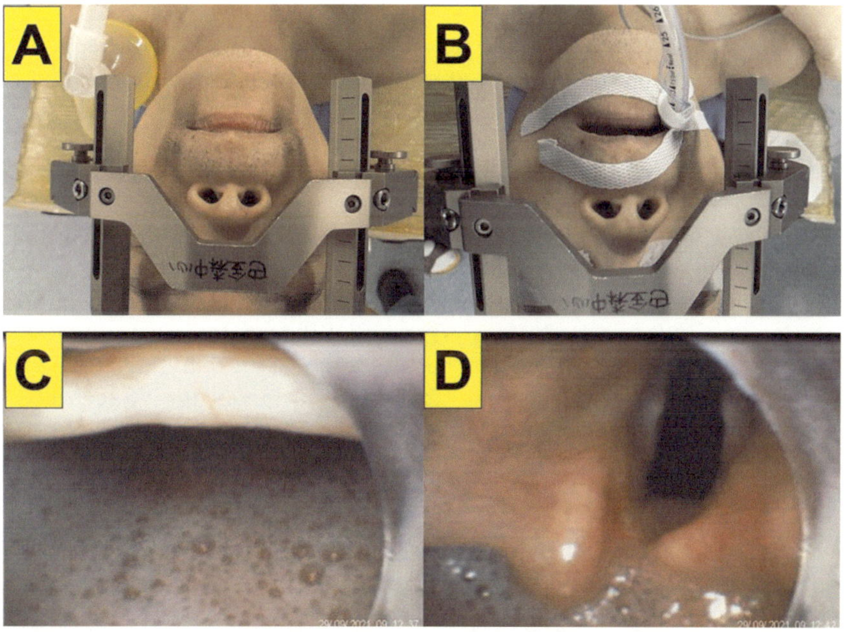

Figure 22.
Application of VS technique in a patient undergoing stereotactic neurosurgery. This 59-year-old man with genetic torsion dystonia and Parkinson's disease (BMI 20.2 kg/m²) underwent frame-based stereotactic procedure for bilateral subthalamus nucleus electrodes implantation. (A) Prior to anesthesia induction, a head frame was mounted and secured. (B) Tracheal intubation was performed with VS technique. (C) Close-up views in front of epiglottis and glottis (D). Copious saliva and secretions were present. The intubation time is 14 s. (Also see the Supplementary Materials Video S21).

use in patients with COVID-19, where this is feasible, and disposable VL blades are preferred" [153]. In reality, for practical reasons, DL was still used in certain cases during the COVID-19 pandemic [154–156].

At the very beginning of the outbreak of COVID-19, it was intuitive to use VL in the management of patients with COVID-19, both in emergent and non-emergent tracheal intubation [157–161]. On the other hand, the safety (transmission rate to the airway managers and team members) and efficacy (e.g., first-pass success rate, intubation time, complications) of VL and DL had not yet been validated in COVID-19 cases [162, 163].

When considering the factors (close proximity of operators and assistants to the patient airway, intubation speed, quality of airway view obtained, or degree of hypoxia during the tracheal intubation) it seems intuitive that VL would be superior to DL (if healthcare resource availability is not an issue). Because of extensive clinical experiences with VS, we applied that technique during the COVID-19 outbreak in Taiwan [65–70]. Since 2020, we have been hit by three outbreak waves (**Figure 23**, time points A, B, and C). From April 2022 to June 2022 22 cases called for tracheal intubation in the negatively pressurized isolation wards and 28 tracheal intubations for emergency surgeries in the negative pressure-operating room. All the tracheal intubations were accomplished with VS technique and a plastic shield (**Figures 24** and **25**). Because our staff (anesthesiologists and residents) are proficient in the use of VS technique (**Table 2**), it seems that COVID-19 intubations did not cause extraordinary mental loading, stress, or technical difficulties for the airway managers.

4.5 Rapid sequence intubation

During the COVID-19 pandemic, it was recommended that PPE be worn by airway managers and airways should be secured in a rapid sequence induction (RSI) or modified RSI [154, 157, 159]. The intubation first-attempt and overall success rates were acceptable. It is inconclusive, however, that RSI itself consistently shows better clinical outcomes than not doing so [164–167]. Moreover, combined use of VL with RSI maneuver does not necessarily shows superiority over DL [168–171].

In our hands, the VS technique provided a higher first-attempt intubation success rate with RSI. The intubation time for VS was non-significantly shorter than DL [73]. Since the benefits of cricoid pressure (CP) is not conclusive, usually we conducted RSI without applying CP. It has been reported that BURP does not help, and jaw-thrust is the most effective maneuver to provide better laryngeal view and shorter intubation time [31]. **Figure 26** shows a tracheal intubation performed using VS technique under RSI protocol. **Figure 27** shows a similar RSI-intubation process in a confirmed COVID-19 positive patient undergoing emergency surgery. In both cases, the intubation process was smooth and swift, and the operators felt safe and better protected against virus exposure.

4.6 Double-lumen endobronchial tube

The clinical role of VL on tracheal intubation with double-lumen endobronchial tube (DLEB tube) for thoracic surgeries has been reviewed [172, 173]. For tracheal intubation with double-lumen endobronchial tube, VL was found either to be superior or equivalent to DL [174–179]. When various outcome parameters were used as comparators (e.g., glottis view, time to intubate, first-pass success rate, complications, ease to use), different types of VL might exhibit their own advantages and

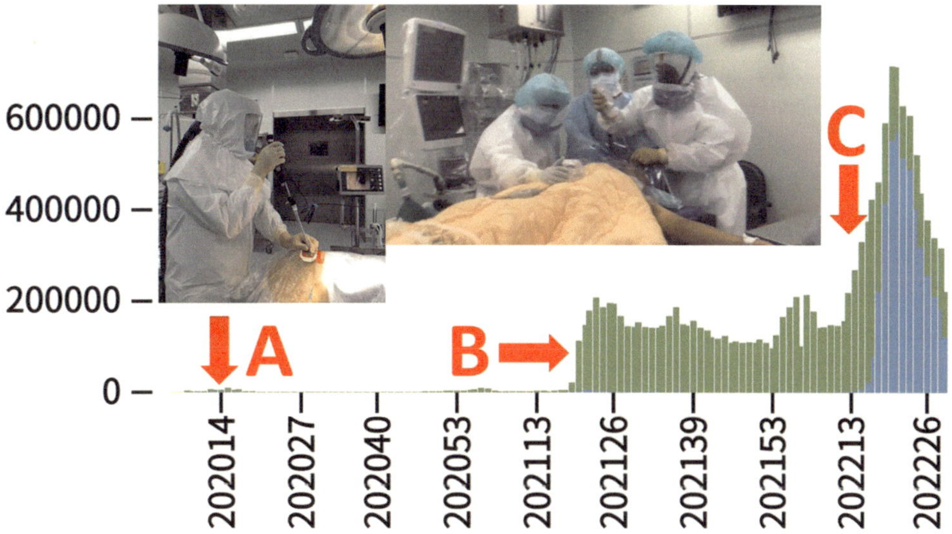

Figure 23.
Application of VS technique to intubate patients at our institute during COVID pandemic in Taiwan. The inset photo (left) shows the operator equipped with PPE intubating with a C-MAC VS (Storz, Germany) in a mannequin simulation model. The inset photo (right) shows the real world when tracheal intubation was conducted with VS technique in an omicron-positive patient. Time point A: February 2020 [65]. Time point B: May 2021 [69]. Time point C: April 2022 [70]. X-axis: The weekly report series number; Y-axis: The patient number. Green and blue colors indicate the surveillance reporting number and confirmed cases number, respectively. Data was modified from Taiwan CDC press release (https://www.cdc.gov.tw/En; data retrieved on July 20, 2022).

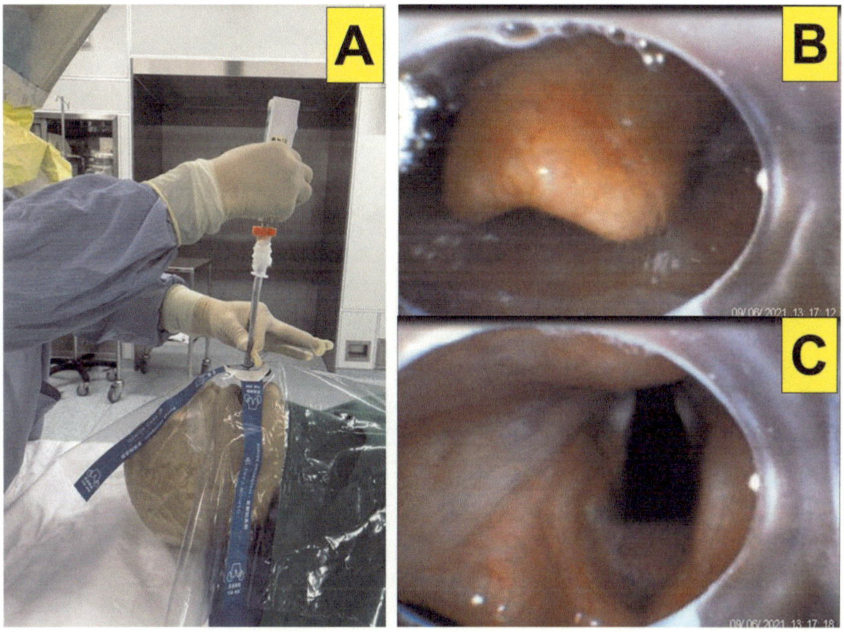

Figure 24.
Combined use of a piece of transparent plastic sheet and VS technique in a mannequin model (A) and in 52-year-old man during COVID-19 pandemic (B and C). The intubation time: 20 s. the detailed technique for this combination method can be seen in the reference [67]. (Also see the Supplementary Materials Video S22).

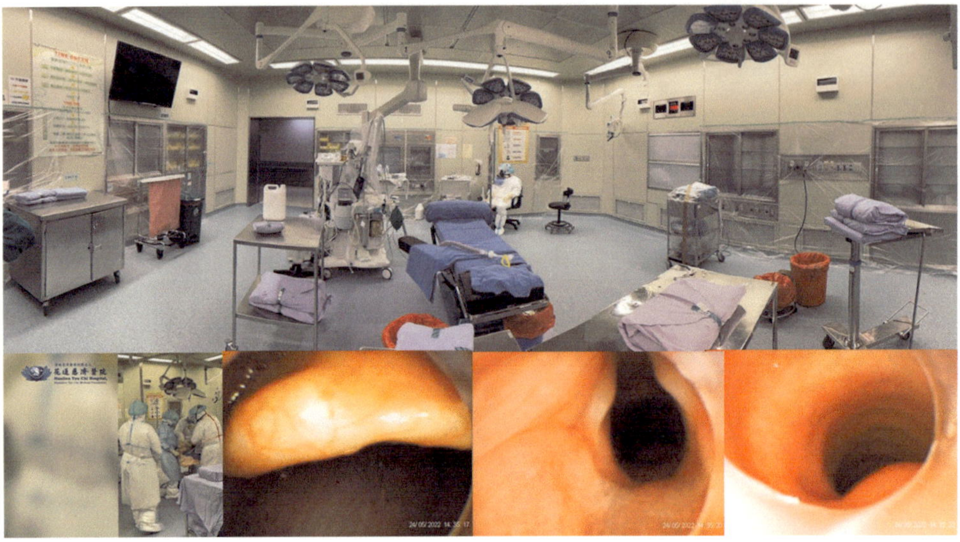

Figure 25.
Combined use of a plastic sheet barrier and VS technique in an omicron-positive patient undergoing emergency neurosurgery for intracerebral hemorrhage. This is a 77-year-old woman (BMI 23.2 kg/m²) with medical history of diabetes and brain tumor. The airway managers wore PPE and a piece of plastic sheet was used as a physical barrier against possible contamination from the patient's airway. The tracheal intubation was smoothly and swiftly achieved with VS technique. The intubation time is 10 s. (Also see the Supplementary Materials Video S23).

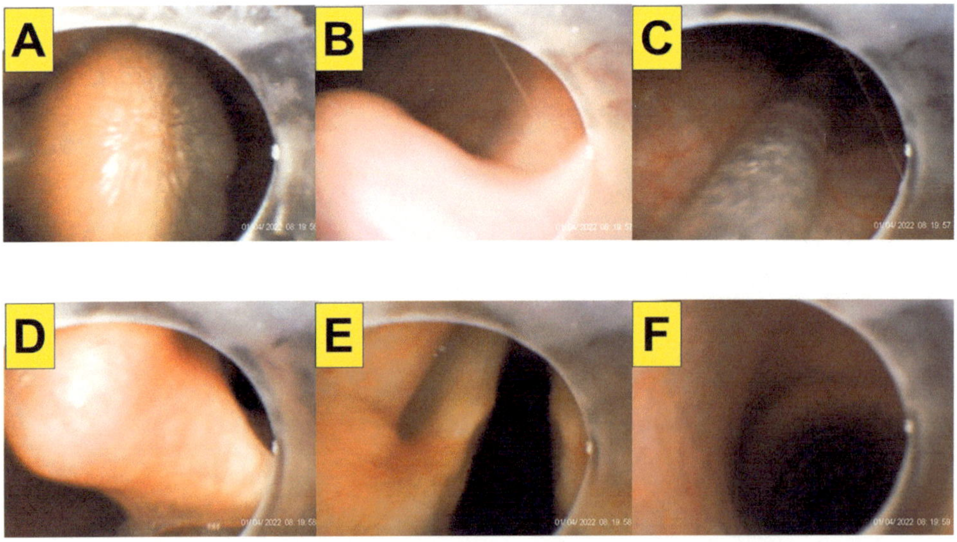

Figure 26.
Application of VS technique with rapid sequence intubation in a patient undergoing emergency abdominal surgery. This 57-year-old man (BMI 26.2 kg/m²) with medical history of duodenal adenocarcinoma (pT4N1) had received a Whipple operation 1 day prior to this emergency surgery. Acute abdominal distention, leukocytosis, and elevated C-reactive protein indicated an intra-abdominal infection. Acute abdominal distention, leukocytosis, and elevated C-reactive protein indicated intra-abdominal infection. Anesthesia induction was conducted using rapid sequence intubation with VS technique. Serial images of oropharynx and larynx (A–C) and glottis-vocal cords-trachea (D–F) are shown. A nasogastric tube is seen in (C). A. The intubation time is 5 s. (Also see the Supplementary Materials Video S24).

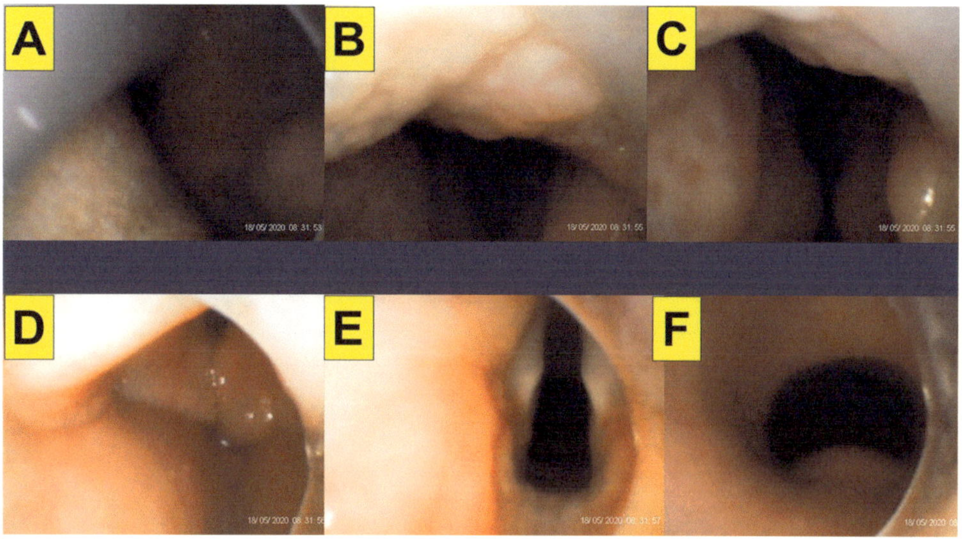

Figure 27.
Application of VS technique with modified rapid sequence intubation in a morbidly obese (BMI 53.3 kg/m², height 150 cm, weight 120 kg) COVID-positive patient undergoing emergency surgery. The intubation time is 7 s. (Also see the Supplementary Materials Video S25).

shortcomings [178, 180]. Not surprisingly, VS technique was alternatively applied for double-lumen endobronchial tube insertion [90, 181, 182]. It was found that VS is quicker, easier, has better glottic visualization, less complications, and was a useful alternative airway tool for placement of DLEB tube. In our single-institute experience, the volume of video-assisted thoracic surgeries using double-lumen endobronchial tube (few using blockers) is about 100 a year. The VS technique has been routinely applied for double-lumen endobronchial tube intubation. **Figure 28** shows such a case. The intubating process is smooth, quick, and with a clear glottis visualization. It should be emphasized that the stick of the VS for DLEB tube intubation should be longer and thinner in order to cope with the design of the DLEB tube.

4.7 Cardiopulmonary resuscitation

It is still a matter of debate whether VL is superior to conventional DL for tracheal intubation during emergency or critical situations. It is generally believed that, if the study outcome parameters are glottis visualization and first-pass success rate, both airway modalities could be equivalent [183–190]. Various factors can come into play including experience, in-hospital/out-of-hospital or emergency room/ICU setting, normal/difficult airway, routine use/rescue alternative, etc. [44, 191–197]. The comparison between VL and DL has been widely conducted [7, 198–202]. Quite often, it was found that VL provides better glottis visualization but does not improve the first-attempt success rate (which is highly experience-dependent) [203]. It is a consensus that uninterrupted, high-quality chest compressions during CPR is crucial to patient outcomes. A "hands-off time" less than 5 s while securing the airway without interruptions of chest compressions during CPR is beneficial for maintaining vital organ perfusion. Meanwhile, during cardiac massage maneuver, it is crucial to avoid unrecognized esophageal intubation [204, 205]. The role of VS has been tested and trained in a mannequin model in the emergency department [206]. Our

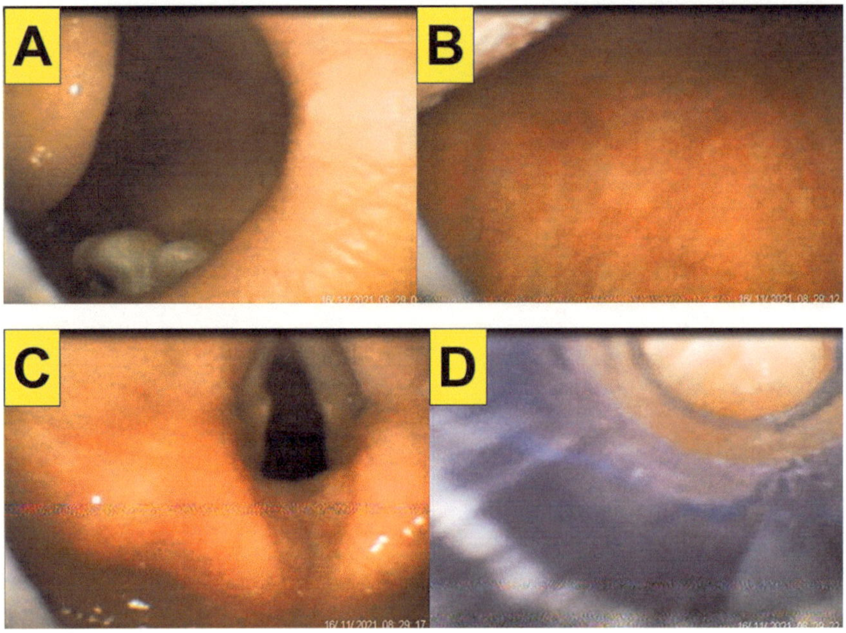

Figure 28.
Application of VS technique for placement of double-lumen endobronchial tube. This is a 71-year-old man (BMI 16.5 kg/m²) who underwent esophageal reconstruction due to esophageal cancer (after definitive concurrent chemoradiotherapy). Although the patient's neck is stiff due to radiation fibrosis, the intubation is 23 s. (Also see the Supplementary Materials Video S26).

single-institute experience is that we always applied VS technique to rescue failed or difficult tracheal intubation in settings outside the operating rooms (e.g., ER, ICU, general wards, endoscopy room). **Figure 29** shows such an example in a 65-year-old man with terminal lung cancer. During the night shift, this patient was found in cardiac arrest and the night staff called code blue but failed to secure the airway after multiple attempts by non-anesthesiologists. Non-stop CPR was continued for 30 min before the anesthesiologist arrived. **Figure 29** shows the tracheal intubation with VS was completed in 6 s without interrupting the CPR course.

5. Pitfalls and tips

5.1 Learning curve for VS technique

It is intuitive to think that DL is a difficult skill to acquire and, VL must be an easier technique for novice trainees to learn. The studies of the learning protocol in normal airway and simulated difficult airway mannequin model usually results in superiority of VL over DL (e.g., better view; shorter intubation times, higher overall success rate, less dental trauma and esophageal intubation) [207–214]. Meanwhile, practicing may improve DL and VL skill competency and the rating of overall ease of use for DL/VL. Opposite learning results (DL faster than VL) in various simulation teaching programs were also reported [215, 216].

The VS technique has been tried in patients with difficult airway related to limited mouth opening [217]. Furthermore, the VS technique has been compared head to head

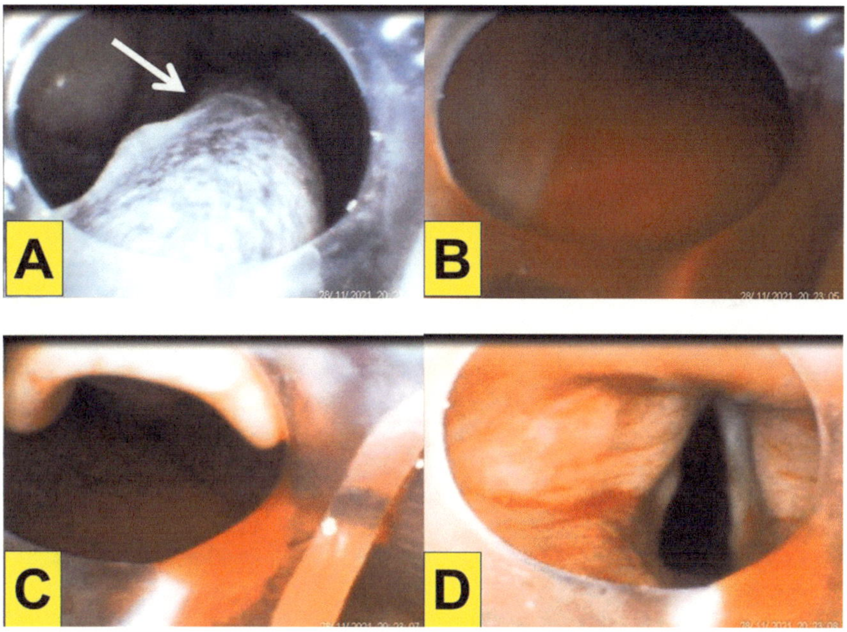

Figure 29.
Application of VS technique for tracheal intubation in a patient who was undergoing cardiopulmonary resuscitation (CPR). This is a 69-year-old man (BMI 24.2 kg/m^2) with lung squamous cell carcinoma and tongue squamous cell carcinoma with metastasis. Neck mobility was limited due to prior tumor-wide excision and neck dissection. Code blue was announced due to massive hemoptysis and in-hospital cardiac arrest in this patient. After repeated attempts of tracheal intubation with VL/DL failed, the airway management rescue team successfully intubated the patient using VS technique while CPR was uninterrupted. The intubation time is 6 s. White arrows denote a suction catheter. (Also see the Supplementary Materials Video S27).

with VL in a normal airway vs. difficult airway due to limited mouth opening mannequin-based study. However, in the difficult airway model, VS was quicker to intubate [149, 218]. Similar results were reported when VS was compared with DL [64, 219, 220]. A semi-rigid VS had the advantages of better maneuverability, superior view of the glottis, and shorter intubation time than a rigid VS. However, when compared with VL in real surgical patients, semi-rigid VS was not superior to VL on intubation time and first-pass success rate [221].

The learning curve for proficiency with optical stylets is reported to be from 10 to 20 uses. In real world experience, we found that the learning curve for performing VS technique by novice trainees (interns and residents) is great. Usually, with a reasonable person standard for these learners, they can accomplish the tracheal intubation task in patients with normal airway. The performance on the task is evaluated by their number of attempts. Usually, the number of trials ranges from 1 to 10 (a steep learning curve). It should be mentioned that our novice trainees always receive structured training courses on cadaver and mannequins before performing on actual patients. **Figures 30** and **31** shows the tracheal intubation with VS technique by an intern.

5.2 Mucus, saliva, secretion, blood

All the optical intubating tools are affected by heavy mucus, secretions, liquid, and gross blood. Simple suctioning is effective in removing these contaminants which easily obscure the optic aperture of the stylet (VS) or scope (VL) and prevent

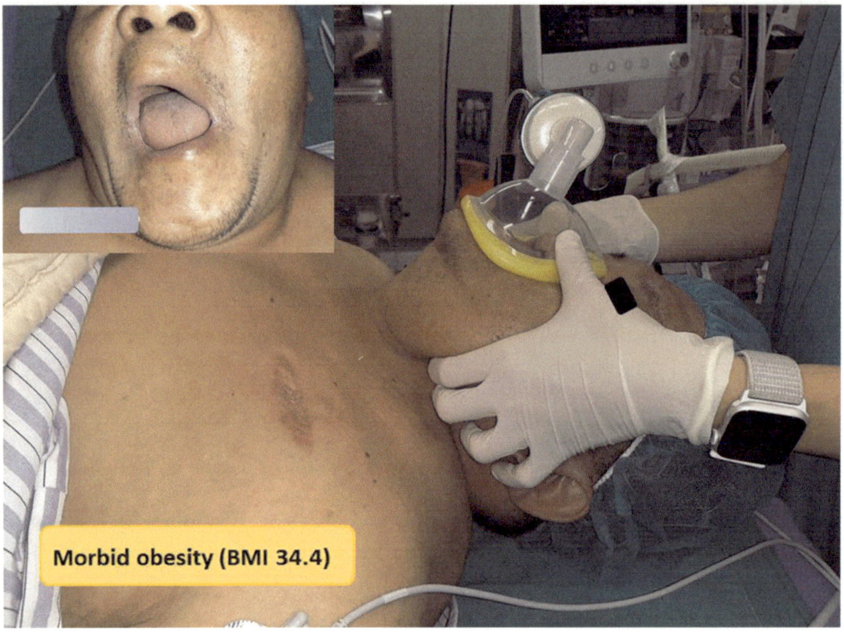

Figure 30.
Application of VS technique for tracheal intubation in a morbidly obese patient (BMI 34.7 kg/m², 167 cm, 97 kg) who underwent percutaneous nephrolithotomy for renal stones. His past medical history includes heart failure due to idiopathic dilated cardiomyopathy, diabetes, hypertension, and he has an implanted cardioverter–defibrillator. Airway management was performed by a competent intern who had a quick learning curve on face mask ventilation and VS technique.

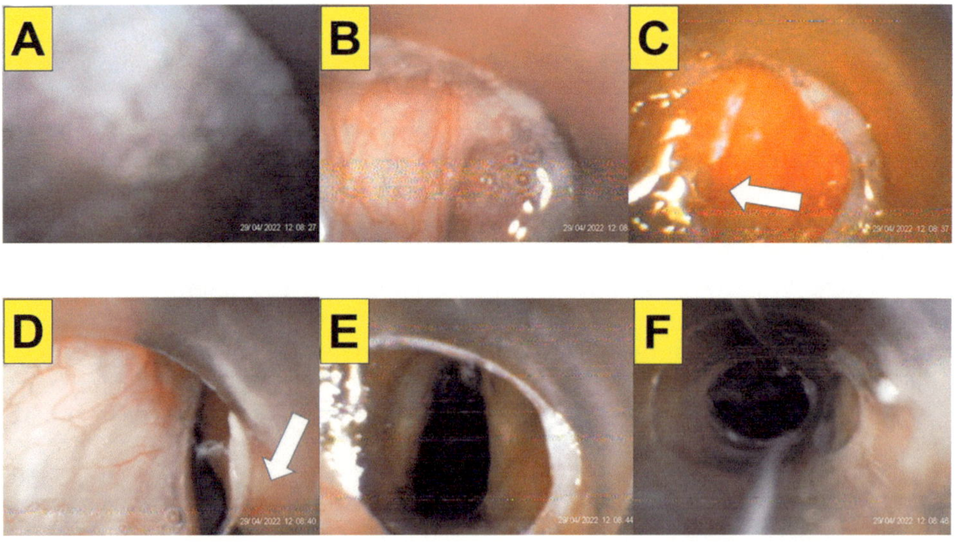

Figure 31.
Application of VS technique for tracheal intubation by a novice trainee (intern). The same patient as in ***Figure 30****. (A) Tongue. (B) Soft tissue. (C) Vallecula (arrow). (D) In front of the epiglottis (arrow). (E) Vocal cords. (F) Entry into trachea. The intubation time is 25 s. Also see the Supplementary Materials Video S28).*

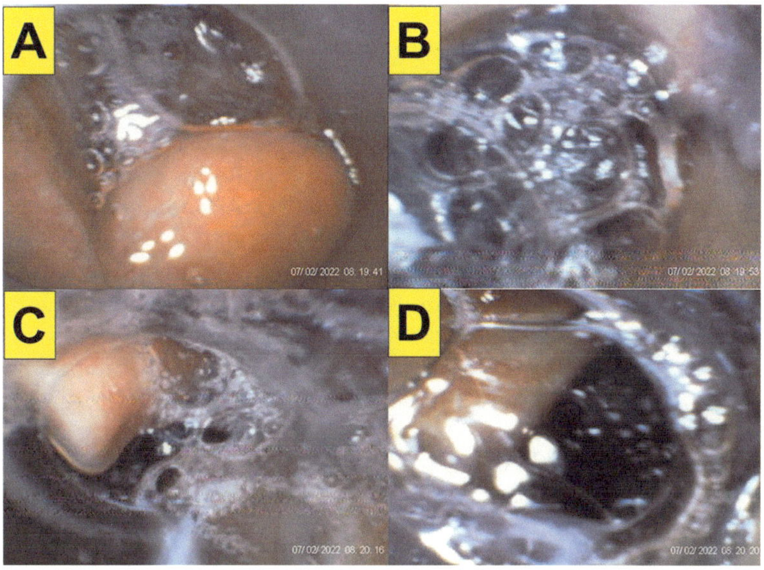

Figure 32.
Application of VS technique for tracheal intubation in a patient with copious secretions in the airway. This is a 65-year-old man with BMI 27.8 kg/m². Prior surgical history included cervical spinal laminoplasty (C4-7 stenosis). The intubation time is 42 s. (Also see the Supplementary Materials Video S29).

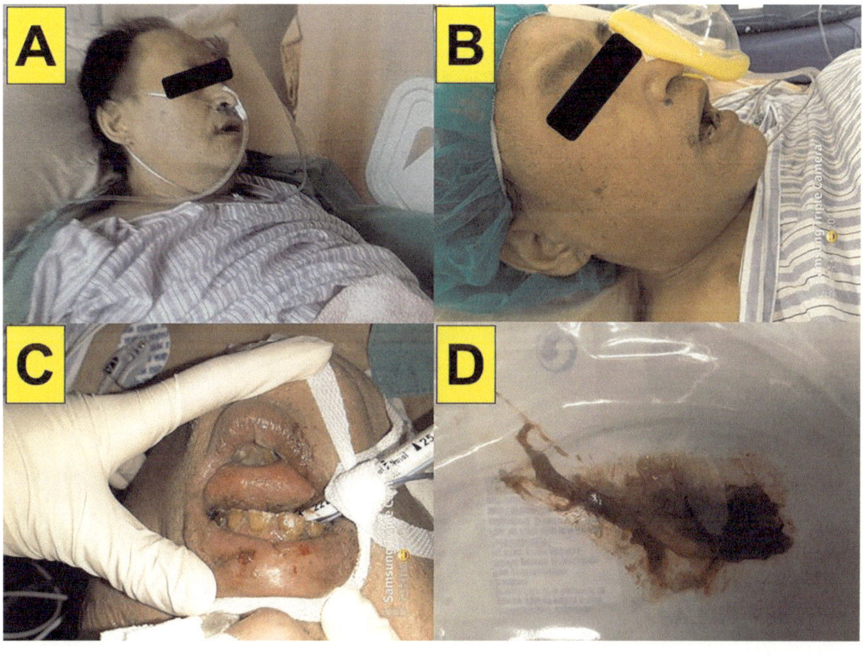

Figure 33.
A case complicated by copious secretions and bleeding during tracheal intubation. This is a 49-year-old man (BMI 31.8 kg/m²) with cirrhosis of liver, pneumonia, and respiratory failure. Debridement was performed for gouty tophi and infection in his extremities. (A) The patient was resting in the ward prior to operation. (B) Before induction of anesthesia. (C) After tracheal intubation was accomplished. (D) Mixture of mucus, saliva, and secretions removed from the patient's airway after intubation.

adequate visualization. In addition to good suctioning, some have proposed that oxygen insufflation will help clear secretions and lead to a better view [222].

Prior to induction of anesthesia, we always ask patients to clear their throat by swallowing any saliva. In addition, if not contraindicated, we would give an anti-sialagogue to reduce the secretions. Usually, this is enough to obtain a clean and clear airway for insertion, advancement, and maneuvering the VS inside of the patient's oropharynx. **Figure 32** shows a patient who had copious secretion during tracheal intubation process.

When patients are bed-ridden or in critical or emergent conditions, it is quite common that they have a significant amount of saliva, mucus, and/or blood in their airways. **Figure 33** shows an unexpected worst-case scenario in a patient in critical condition. Prior to VS, it was not recognized that the patient had a huge amount of mixed secretions, mucus, and blood in his oropharynx. When the picture obtained from VS optical lens appeared onto the video screen, nothing was easily identified (**Figure 34**). We were still able to navigate in the oropharyngeal space and advanced the stylet into the glottis eventually (**Figure 34**). In the same patient, after his airway was secured by VS, it was still a struggle to clear the copious secretions to obtain a view by VL of the glottis and ET tube (**Figure 35**).

There are occasional cases with head and neck cancer where FOB is advisable over VS. In such a patient with laryngeal cancer who had received multiple radiation therapies, the mouth opening was limited, the neck was stiff, and the hypopharynx and glottis were swollen (**Figures 36** and **37**). VS was tried after induction of anesthesia (**Figure 38**). However, copious mucus, secretions, and saliva seriously obscured the visualization of the spotted optic lens on the VS. The epiglottis could not be lifted up at all. The airway

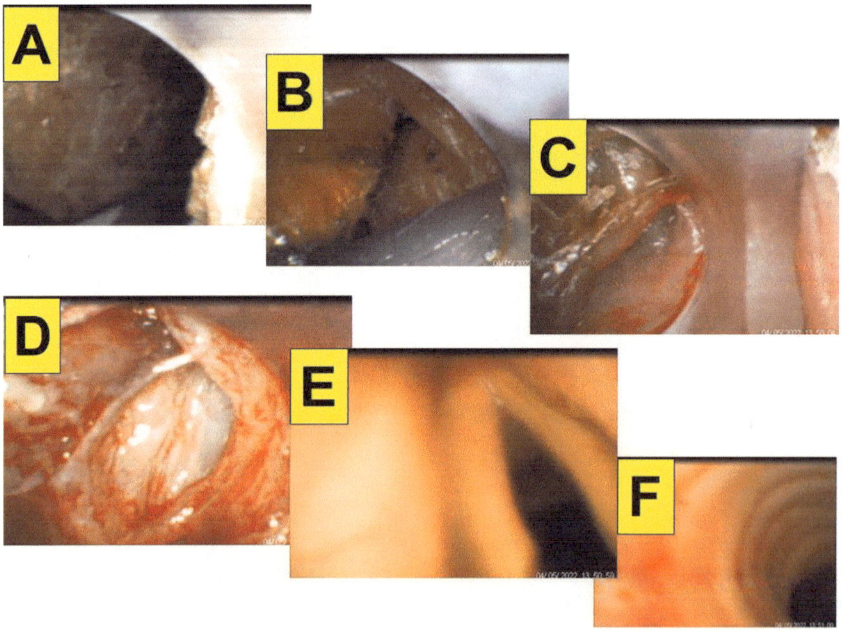

Figure 34.
*A case complicated by copious secretions and bleeding during tracheal intubation. The same patient as in **Figures 33** and **35**. Serial close-up view from VS camera. A bunch of mucus and blood mixtures were seen and blocked the view for advancement of the stylet (A–D). After struggling, a clear glottis view was eventually obtained (E) and ET tube was successfully secured into trachea (F). The intubation time is 80 s. (Also see the Supplementary Materials Video S30).*

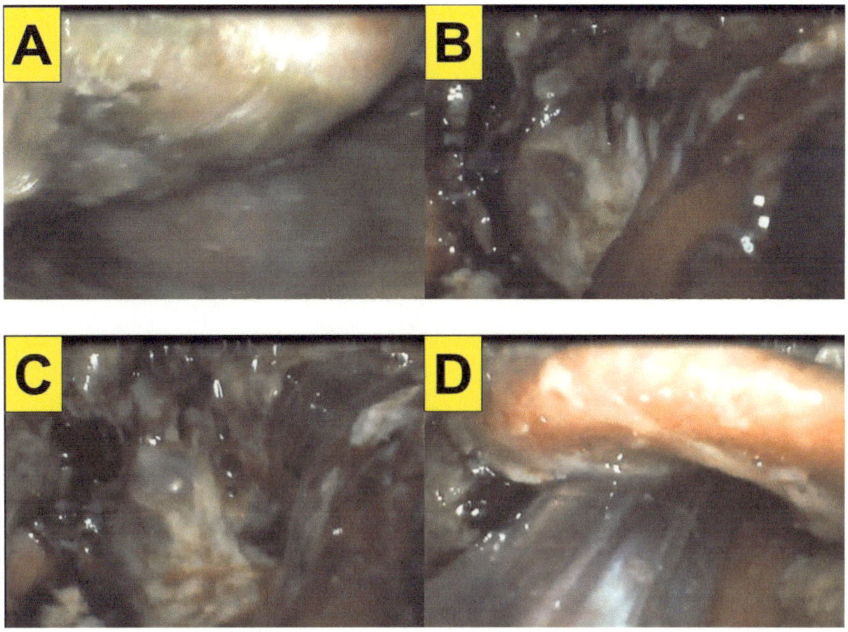

Figure 35.
A case complicated by copious secretions and bleeding during tracheal intubation (the same patient as in ***Figures 33*** *and* ***34****). After airway secured by VS, VL was used to examine patient's airway. (A–C) Serial close-up views from VL camera show a bunch of mucus and blood mixtures blocking the view in the patient's airway. (D) After adequate suction, the views became clearer. (Also see the Supplementary Materials Video S31).*

was eventually secured with FOB (**Figure 39**). **Figure 40** shows the intubation images of the same patient during his elective tracheostomy 3 weeks later. Tracheal intubation was performed by FOB. This extreme clinical case should be regarded as the limit of using VS technique in comparison to the conventional role of FOB.

5.3 Video-video paired technique

Combined use of DL/VL with FOB has been a common alternative in certain anticipated difficult airways [223–231]. Similarly, it has also been thought to combine VL and a particular shaped stylet (or bougie-kind of introducer). When lighted or optical stylets became available, it was natural to combine both for tracheal intubation in scenarios like ankylosing spondylitis, morbid obesity, or certain congenital anomalies involving orofacial or head/neck regions. Using an appropriate videolaryngoscopic blade may create better oropharyngeal space and laryngeal views and therefore may reduce stylet use in patients with normal airway [8], but not replace stylet use in morbidly obese patients [123].

In a patient with a difficult airway, after several attempts at laryngoscopy had failed, endotracheal intubation was accomplished by the combined use of a laryngoscope and the Bonfils rigid fiberscope [232, 233]. This successful combo technique involved two airway managers. One used a laryngoscope to displace the patient's tongue to the left ventral part of the mouth and cleared the airway by suctioning. The other one inserted the Bonfils rigid fiberscope, followed the blade of the laryngoscope to the larynx, obtained a good view of the vocal cords, and railroaded the ET tube into the trachea. It was reported the intubation time was 20 s. Although it was not known

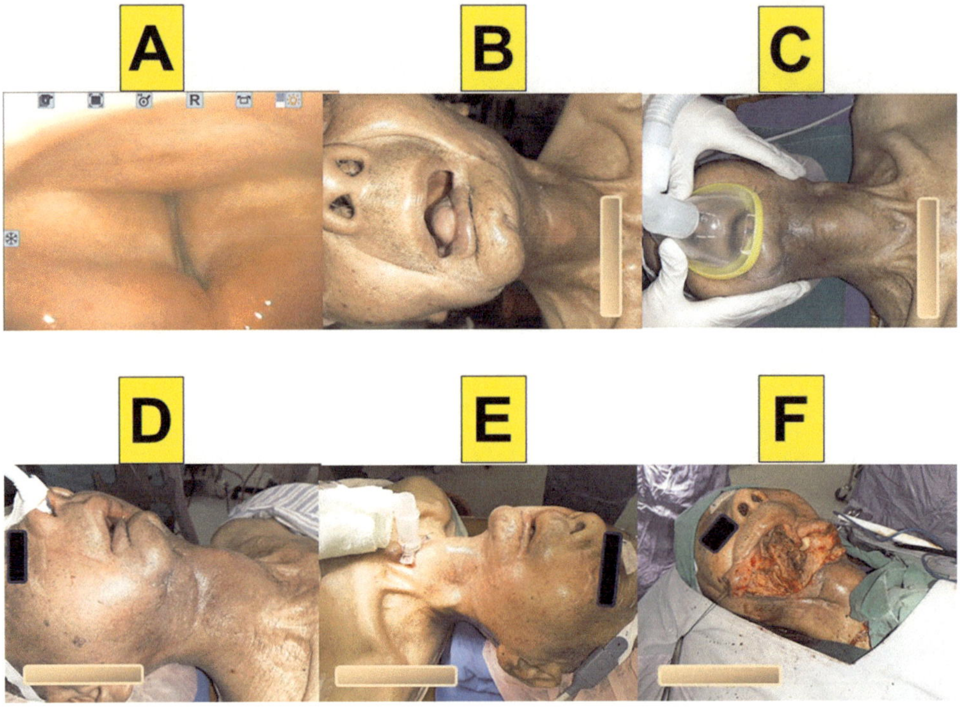

Figure 36.
An extreme and anticipated difficult airway in a patient with mandibular sarcoma. Repeated surgical treatments (tumor wide excision, neck dissection, mandibulectomy, free flap reconstruction) and concurrent chemoradiotherapy were performed. (A) Pre-operative endoscopic examination showed swollen glottis. (B, C) Limited mouth opening and stiff neck due to radiation therapy. The face mask ventilation was adequate to maintain oxygenation. (D) After nasal tracheal intubation using fiberoptic intubation. (E) After tracheostomy. (F) During surgery.

the exact underlying cause for the several failed attempts at laryngoscopy in this patient, successful rescue with VS in 20 s is reasonably acceptable.

The shape of the stylet may affect the effectiveness and performance of VL in patients with normal airways [234]. The combined use of VS and VL has been helpful in patients with normal [235] and difficult airways [14, 34, 35, 236]. While VS has been used as an adjunct to DL/VL, we prefer to reverse the ancillary relationship between VS and VL/DL. Namely, we proposed the DL/VL play an adjunct to VS. The role of DL/VL is to open the airway, create minimal oropharyngeal space, lift up the epiglottis, and finally allow VS to pass through under the epiglottis and acquire a better glottis view. It is worthy to mention that this combination method (VS-VL) has been applied in many difficult cases at our institute. One example involves a patient with mucopolysaccharidosis (MPS) who also had prior C-spine surgery and was receiving a corneal transplantation. He had a limited mouth-opening and flaccid epiglottis which could not be lifted up by jaw-thrust maneuver at all. However, with the aid of VL, tracheal intubation was smooth and swift with VS technique. Another case involved a morbidly obese patient (BMI 56 and 60) who underwent two separate operations (UPPP and bariatric surgery) at our institution. Several attempts at tracheal intubation with various intubation tools failed. With the aid of VL, tracheal intubation was eventually accomplished by VS technique without complications.

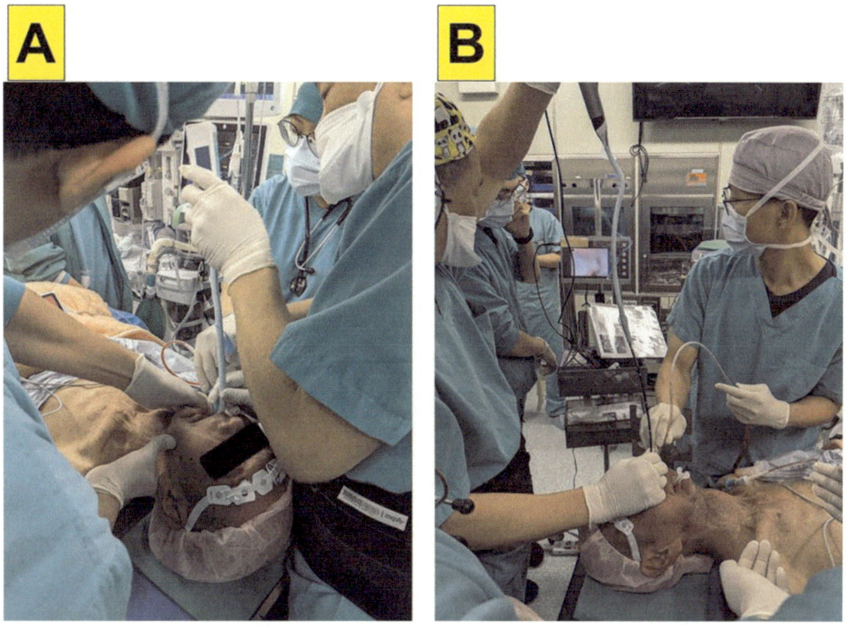

Figure 37.
*Adoption of VS (A) and FOB (B) in the same patient as in **Figures 36–40**. It is noted that, after failure of VS technique, FOB was used to establish nasal tracheal intubation.*

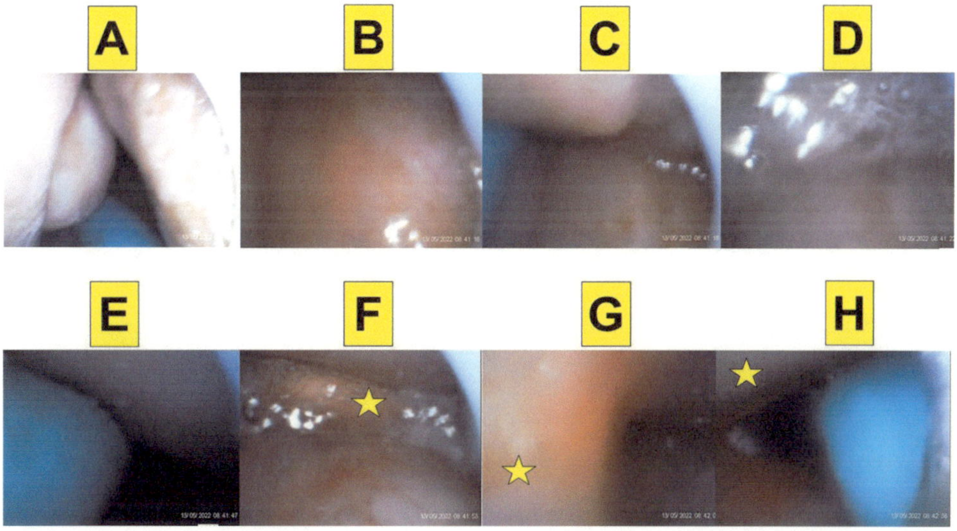

Figure 38.
*Serial views from VS camera during tracheal intubation (same patient in **Figures 36–40**). (A–C) The oropharynx was crowded due to radiation fibrosis of the neck. (D–F) Copious secretions and saliva were noted. The epiglottis (labeled by the yellow star) was firmly attached to the posterior pharyngeal wall when the patient was anesthetized and paralyzed (E–H). The maneuverability of the VS was seriously hindered by the limited mouth opening and rigid neck. Intubation failed after several attempts.*

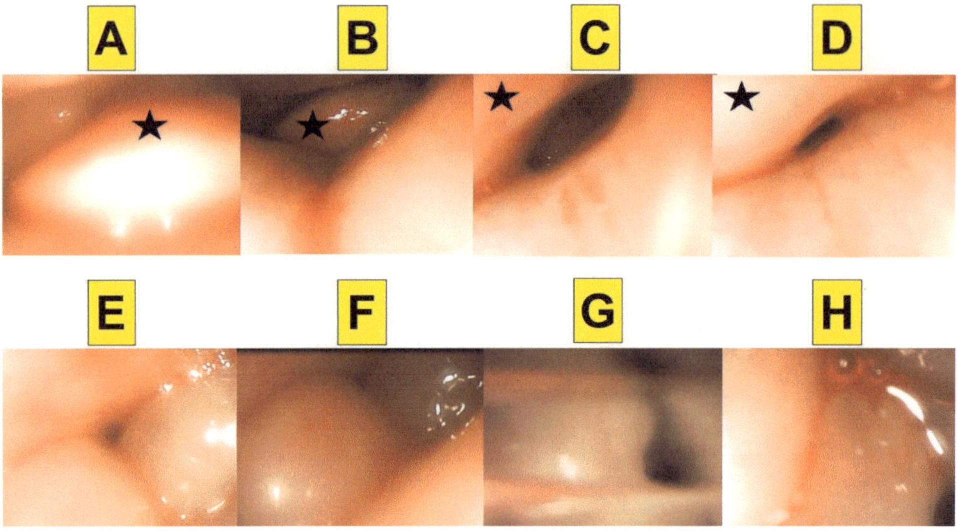

Figure 39.
Rescued intubation with FOB when the patient's controlled ventilation was reverted back to spontaneous respiration. (A–D) The epiglottis (labeled by the black star) was firmly attached to the posterior pharyngeal wall. (C, D) There appeared a tiny slit only when the patient exhaled. The airway operator then took this chance to sneak the FOB tip through this tiny slit and passed under the epiglottis. Subsequent views of swollen glottis (E, F) and vocal cords (G, H). Same patient as in ***Figures 36–40****.*

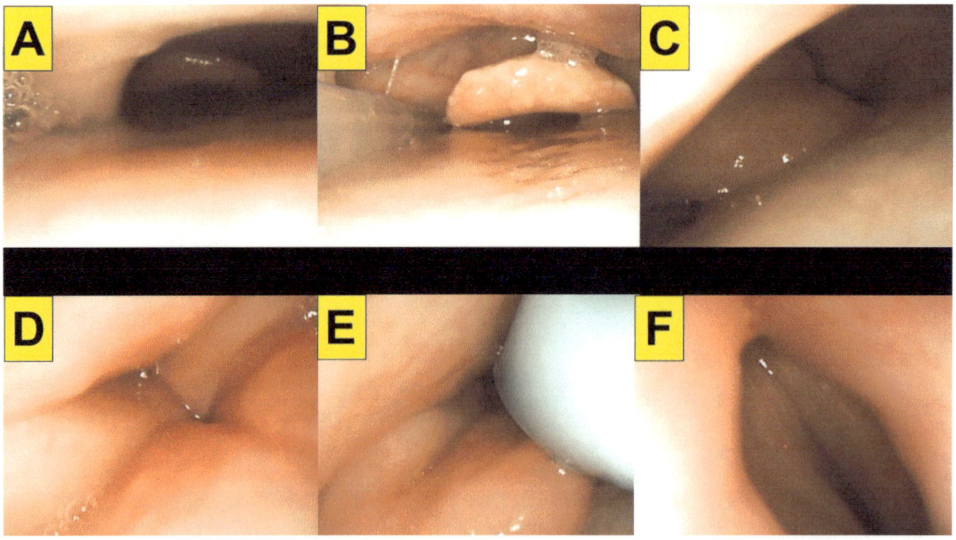

Figure 40.
Awake FOB under light sedation was performed in the same patient 3 weeks later. Elective tracheostomy was scheduled because it became progressively more difficult for the patient to breathe. (A, B) The epiglottis was lying against the posterior pharyngeal wall and there was a very narrow space to allow air to breathe out. A nasogastric feeding tube was seen. (C) A partial view of glottis under the epiglottis. (D) View of closed vocal cords. (E) The tip of a suction catheter was seen and it was withdrawn back later. (F) Vocal cords was in the closed status before the fiber's entry into trachea. Same patient as in ***Figures 36–40****.*

In contrast to previous experiences of using the combined VS/VL technique in difficult airway clinical scenarios [34, 35] and in mannequin models [237], we have routinely applied this technique in normal airways in our daily practice. Included among our routine use of VS-VL for daily practice are cases of intraoperative neurophysiologic monitoring (IONM) during thyroidectomy [238]. The IONM allows confirmation of the functional integrity of the recurrent laryngeal nerve as well as facilitates identification of the RLN before visualization during operations. While VS technique provides an accurate and swift tracheal intubation (e.g., especially in the presence of a giant goiter), VL ensures the contact surface of a specialized EMG endotracheal tube (e.g., Xomed and TriVantage Nerve Integrity Monitoring (NIM) ETTs, Medtronic Xomed Inc., Jacksonville, FL, USA) can been seen and placed in the correct spot between the vocal cords.

Here we demonstrate two cases of using the VS-VL paired technique in patients with normal airways during our routine practice. **Figures 41** and **42** shows a patient with a flat epiglottis and **Figures 43** and **44** shows another patient with an omega-shape epiglottis. Neither epiglottis prevented the convenience and ease of using VS-VL paired technique to intubate.

6. Future perspectives

VL for tracheal intubation has been the norm for tracheal intubation for several decades [50, 239]. Since the introduction of the Shikani video-associated stylet technique for intubation in 1999 [6], numerous commercially available video-assisted

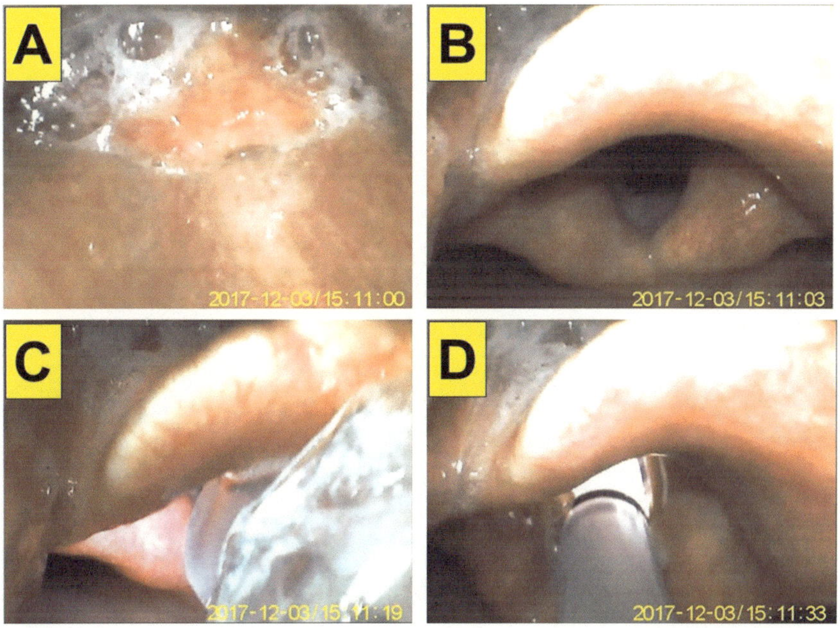

Figure 41.
*Video-video paired technique for tracheal intubation. This is a 68-year-old man with BMI 25.9 kg/m^2. Vitrectomy was scheduled for recurrent total retinal detachment. VL was used as an adjunct to VS. (A) A flat epiglottis. (B) Cormack-Lehane grade IIa. (C) Passage of the VS stylet-ET tube into vocal cords. (D) Entry of the ET tube into trachea. The same patient as in **Figure 42**. (Also see the Supplementary Materials Video S32).*

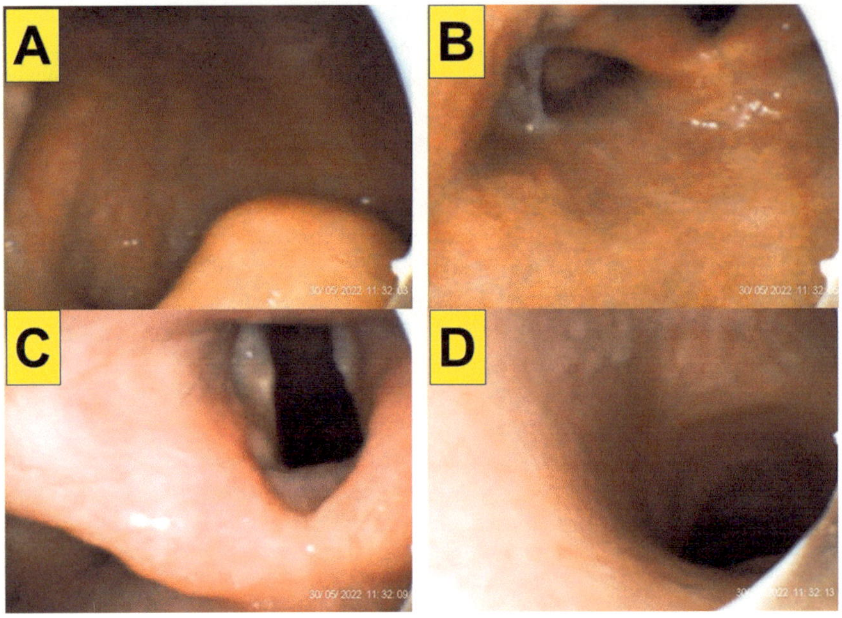

Figure 42.
Views from VS camera. The same patient as in ***Figure 41****. After glottis views were obtained by VL, the VS was inserted and advanced. (A) Oropharynx. (B) Larynx. LQS score grade 1. (C) Full glottis view. (D) Entry into trachea. It is noted that, with the help of VL, the airway is wide open and a perfect glottis view is easy to obtain. The intubation time is 14 s. (Also see the Supplementary Materials Video S33).*

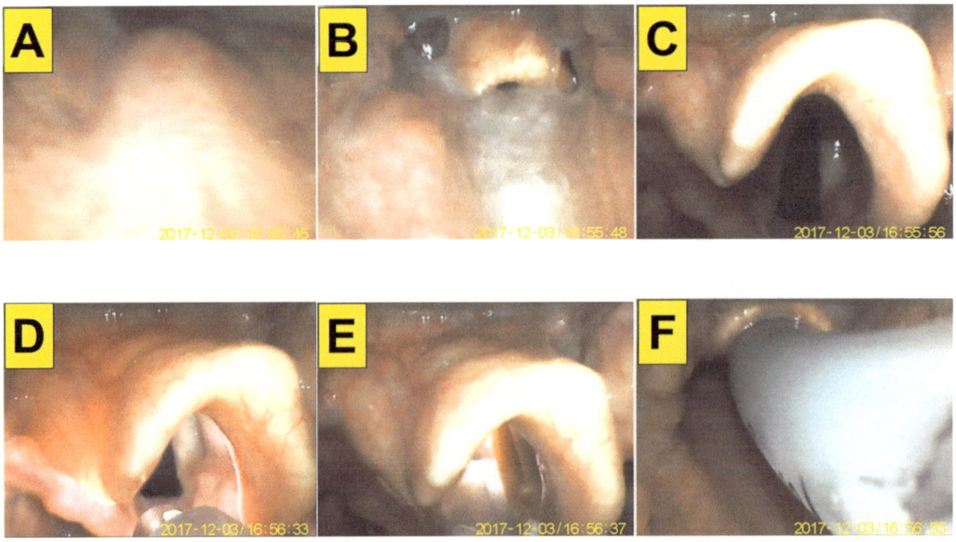

Figure 43.
Video-video paired technique for tracheal intubation. This 68-year-old man (BMI 26.8 kg/m²) underwent a bipolar hemiarthroplasty due to femoral neck fracture. Past history includes lung adenocarcinoma and cervical spine stenosis (C3-6). VL was used as an adjunct to VS. (A) Uvula. (B–E) An omega-shaped epiglottis. (C) Cormack-Lehane grade I. (D, E) Passage of the VS stylet-ET tube into vocal cords. (F) Entry of the ET tube into trachea. The same patient as in ***Figure 44****. (Also see the Supplementary Materials Video S34).*

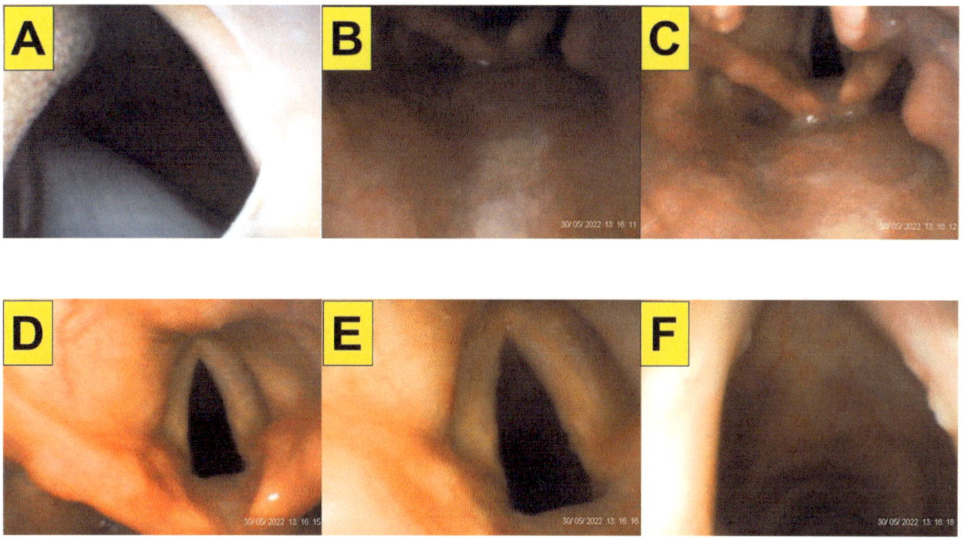

Figure 44.
*Views from VS camera. The same patient as in **Figure 43**. After glottis views were obtained by VL, the VS was inserted and advanced. (A) Oropharynx. (B, C) Larynx. LQS score grade 1. (D, E) Full glottis view. (F) Entry into trachea. The intubation time is 15 s. (Also see the Supplementary Materials Video S35).*

intubating stylet products have been brought to market. Some of the advantages of the VS technique include maneuverability, better visualization, the ability to negotiate a confined oropharyngeal space, the ability to avoid any trauma to the airway or the teeth, ease of use, and affordability. A high first-attempt success rate, shorter intubation time, and less trauma are additional advantages which lead to less autonomic stimulation. These advantages are why VS has been overwhelmingly accepted and the most prevalent intubating tool in Taiwan since 2016. We hope that this review article will educate intubation providers from various regions of the world and make VS accepted universally. It is still to be determined whether VS will become a first-line technique in the airway guidelines for routine intubations, or whether it will be restricted to more challenging airways situations.

7. Conclusion

In this review article, we presented the application of the Shikani video-assisted stylet technique for intubation in various clinical scenarios and practice settings. In our experience, VS has proved to be an effective and sometimes invaluable method for managing both normal and difficult airways.

Acknowledgements

The author (HN Luk) acknowledged the full support from Hualien Tzuchi Medical Center, Hualien, Taiwan. Special thanks to Professor Dr. Shinn-Zong Lin, MD, PhD, CPI, Fellow of AAAS and AANS.

The authors declare no conflict of interest. Written informed consents were obtained from all the patients (or their legally authorized representatives) for the use of their clinical data in this review article. Patient's privacy and data confidentiality were protected in compliance with the Declaration of Helsinki and local human research ethics regulations.

Author details

Hsiang-Ning Luk[1,2*], Hsuan-Nu Luk[3], Jason Zhensheng Qu[4] and Alan Shikani[5,6]

1 Department of Anesthesia, Hualien Tzuchi Hospital, Hualien, Taiwan

2 Bio-Math Laboratory, Department of Financial Engineering, Providence University, Taichung, Taiwan

3 Department of Medicine, School of Medicine, Beijing University, Beijing, China

4 Department of Anesthesia, Critical Care and Pain Medicine, Massachusetts General Hospital, Harvard Medical School, Boston, MA, USA

5 Division of Otolaryngology-Head and Neck Surgery, LifeBridge Sinai Hospital, Baltimore, MD, USA

6 Division of Otolaryngology-Head and Neck Surgery, MedStar Union Memorial Hospital, Baltimore, MD, USA

*Address all correspondence to: lukairforce@gmail.com

References

[1] Jephcott A. The Macintosh laryngoscope. A historical note on its clinical and commercial development. Anaesthesia. 1984;**39**:474-479. DOI: 10.1111/j.1365-2044.1984.tb07319.x

[2] Pieters BM, Eindhoven GB, Acott C, van Zundert AA. Pioneers of laryngoscopy: Indirect, direct and video laryngoscopy. Anaesthesia and Intensive Care. 2015;**43**(Suppl):4-11. DOI: 10.1177/0310057X150430S103

[3] Katz RL, Berci G. The optical stylet—A new intubation technique for adults and children with specific reference to teaching. Anesthesiology. 1979;**51**: 251-254

[4] Berci G, Katz R. Optical stylet: An aid to intubation and teaching. The Annals of Otology, Rhinology, and Laryngology. 1979;**88**:828-831

[5] Bonfils P. Difficult intubation in Pierre-Robin children, a new method: The retromolar route. Der Anaesthesist. 1983;**32**:363-367 (in German) PMID: 6614426

[6] Shikani AH. New "seeing" stylet-scope and method for the management of the difficult airway. Otolaryngology and Head and Neck Surgery. 1999;**120**: 113-116. DOI: 10.1016/S0194-5998(99) 70380-3

[7] Hansel J, Rogers AM, Lewis SR, Cook TM, Smith AF. Videolaryngoscopy versus direct laryngoscopy for adults undergoing tracheal intubation. Cochrane Library: Cochrane Reviews. 2022;**4**(4):CD011136. DOI: 10.1002/14651858.CD011136.pub3

[8] van Zundert A, Maassen R, Lee R, Willems R, Timmerman M, Siemonsma M, et al. A Macintosh laryngoscope blade for videolaryngoscopy reduces stylet use in patients with normal airways. Anesthesia and Analgesia. 2009;**109**:825-831. DOI: 10.1213/ane.0b013e3181ae39db

[9] Greenland KB. A proposed model for direct laryngoscopy and tracheal intubation. Anaesthesia. 2008;**63**: 156-161. DOI: 10.1111/j.1365-2044.2007.05326.x

[10] Lee L, Weightman WM. Laryngoscopy force in the sniffing position compared to the extension-extension position. Anaesthesia. 2008; **63**:375-378. DOI: 10.1111/j.1365-2044.2008.05492.x

[11] El-Orbany M, Woehlck H, Salem MR. Head and neck position for direct laryngoscopy. Anesthesia and Analgesia. 2011;**113**:103-109. DOI: 10.1213/ANE.0b013e31821c7e9c

[12] Liem EB, Bjoraker DG, Gravenstein D. New options for airway management: Intubating fibreoptic stylets. British Journal of Anaesthesia. 2003;**91**:408-418. DOI: 10.1093/bja/aeg011

[13] Evans A, Morris S, Petterson J, Hall JE. A comparison of the seeing optical stylet and the gum elastic bougie in simulated difficult tracheal intubation: A manikin study. Anaesthesia. 2006;**61**:478-481. DOI: 10.1111/j.1365-2044.2006.04539.x

[14] Kovacs G, Law AJ, Petrie D. Awake fiberoptic intubation using an optical stylet in an anticipated difficult airway. Annals of Emergency Medicine. 2007; **49**:81-83. DOI: 10.1016/j.annemergmed.2006.03.024

[15] Komatsu R, Kamata K, Hamada K, Sessler DI, Ozaki M. Airway scope and

StyletScope for tracheal intubation in a simulated difficult airway. Anesthesia and Analgesia. 2009;**108**:273-279. DOI: 10.1213/ane.0b013e3181 8a4398

[16] Cohen SM, Laurito CE, Segil LJ. Examination of the hypopharynx predicts ease of laryngoscopic visualization and subsequent intubation: A prospective study of 665 patients. Journal of Clinical Anesthesia. 1992;**4**: 310-314. DOI: 10.1016/0952-8180(92) 90136-o

[17] Rose DK, Cohen MM. The airway: Problems and predictions in 18,500 patients. Canadian Journal of Anaesthesia. 1994;**41**:372-383. DOI: 10.1007/BF03009858

[18] Tremblay MH, Williams S, Robitaille A, Drolet P. Poor visualization during direct laryngoscopy and high upper lip bite test score are predictors of difficult intubation with the GlideScope® videolaryngoscope. Anesthesia and Analgesia. 2008;**106**: 1495-1500. DOI: 10.1213/ane.0b013 e318168b38f

[19] Cormack RS, Lehane J. Difficult tracheal intubation in obstetrics. Anaesthesia. 1984;**39**:1105-1111 PMID: 6507827

[20] Wilson ME, Spiegelhalter D, Robertson JA, Lesser P. Predicting difficult intubation. British Journal of Anaesthesia. 1988;**61**:211-216. DOI: 10.1093/bja/61.2.211

[21] Levitan RM, Ochroch EA, Kush S, Shofer FS, Hollander JE. Assessment of airway visualization: Validation of the percentage of glottic opening (POGO) scale. Academic Emergency Medicine. 1998;**5**:919-923. DOI: 10.1111/ j.1553-2712.1998.tb02823.x

[22] Ochroch EA, Hollander JE, Kush S, Shofer FS, Levitan RM. Assessment of laryngeal view: Percentage of glottic opening score vs Cormack and Lehane grading. Canadian Journal of Anaesthesia. 1999;**46**:987-990. DOI: 10.1007/BF03013137

[23] Xue FS, Liu JH, Yuan YJ, Wang Q, Liao X. Oxygen flush is an effective means to eliminate obscured vision by fogging during intubation using the Airtraq(®) optical laryngoscope. Canadian Journal of Anaesthesia. 2010; **57**:1133-1135. DOI: 10.1007/s12630-010-9389-y

[24] Thong SY, Wong TG. Clinical uses of the Bonfils retromolar intubation fiberscope: A review. Anesthesia and Analgesia. 2012;**115**:855-866. DOI: 10.1213/ANE.0b013e3182 65bae2

[25] Haba M, Komasawa N. A simple method for preventing the fog in the videolaryngoscope monitor during awake intubation. Journal of Clinical Anesthesia. 2018;**44**:84-85. DOI: 10.1016/j.jclinane.2017.11.013

[26] Park JW, Choi HJ. Study on the effect of a cold environment on the quality of three video laryngoscopes: McGrath MAC, GlideScope ranger, and Pentax airway scope. Clinical and Experimental Emergency Medicine. 2019;**6**:351-355. DOI: 10.15441/ ceem.18.063

[27] Dean P, Kerrey B. Video screen visualization patterns when using a video laryngoscope for tracheal intubation: A systematic review. Journal of the American College of Emergency Physicians Open. 2022;**3**(1):e12630. DOI: 10.1002/emp2.12630

[28] Agrò F, Cataldo R, Carassiti M, Costa F. The seeing stylet: A new device

for tracheal intubation. Resuscitation. 2000;**44**:177-180. DOI: 10.1016/s0300-9572(00)00137-4

[29] Biro P, Weiss M, Gerber A, Pasch T. Comparison of a new video-optical intubation stylet versus the conventional malleable stylet in simulated difficult tracheal intubation. Anaesthesia. 2000; **55**:886-889. DOI: 10.1046/j.1365-A2044.2000.01519.x

[30] Pfitzner L, Cooper MG, Ho D. The Shikani seeing stylet for difficult intubation in children: Initial experience. Anaesthesia and Intensive Care. 2002;**30**: 462-466. DOI: 10.1177/0310057X0203000411

[31] Phua DS, Mah CL, Wang CF. The Shikani optical stylet as an alternative to the GlideScope® videolaryngoscope in simulated difficult intubations—A randomised controlled trial. Anaesthesia. 2012;**67**:402-406. DOI: 10.1111/j.1365-2044.2011.07023.x

[32] Lee AR, Yang S, Shin YH, Kim JA, Chung IS, Cho HS, et al. A comparison of the BURP and conventional and modified jaw thrust manoeuvres for orotracheal intubation using the Clarus video system. Anaesthesia. 2013;**68**:931-937. DOI: 10.1111/anae.12282

[33] Yang SM, Kim H, Chang JE, Min SW, Lee JM, Hwang JY. A comparison of single-handed chin lift and two-handed jaw thrust for tracheal intubation using a lightwand. Journal of Anesthesia. 2017;**31**:5-10. DOI: 10.1007/s00540-016-2276-0

[34] van Zundert AA, Pieters BM. Combined technique using videolaryngoscopy and Bonfils for a difficult airway intubation. British Journal of Anaesthesia. 2012;**108**: 327-328. DOI: 10.1093/bja/aer471

[35] Chen WC, Lin S, He HF. Case report: Double visualization intubation strategy for patients with ankylosing spondylitis. Frontiers of Medicine (Lausanne). 2022; **9**:659624. DOI: 10.3389/fmed.2022.659624

[36] Krage R, van Rijn C, van Groeningen D, Loer SA, Schwarte LA, Schober P. Cormack-Lehane classification revisited. British Journal of Anaesthesia. 2010;**105**:220-227. DOI: 10.1093/bja/aeq136

[37] Pearce AC, Duggan LV, El-Boghdadly K. Making the grade: Has Cormack and Lehane grading stood the test of time? Anaesthesia. 2021;**76**: 705-709. DOI: 10.1111/anae.15446

[38] Cook TM, Boniface NJ, Seller C, Hughes J, Damen C, MacDonald L, et al. Universal videolaryngoscopy: A structured approach to conversion to videolaryngoscopy for all intubations in an anaesthetic and intensive care department. British Journal of Anaesthesia. 2018;**120**:173-180. DOI: 10.1016/j.bja.2017.11.014

[39] Lascarrou JB, Boisrame-Helms J, Bailly A, Le Thuaut A, Kamel T, Mercier E, Ricard JD, et al; Clinical Research in Intensive Care and Sepsis (CRICS) Group. Video laryngoscopy vs direct laryngoscopy on successful first-pass orotracheal intubation among ICU patients: A randomized clinical trial. Journal of the American Medical Association 2017;**317**:483-493. DOI: 10.1001/jama.2016.20603.

[40] Cormack RS. Cormack-Lehane classification revisited. British Journal of Anaesthesia. 2010;**105**:867-868. DOI: 10.1093/bja/aeq324

[41] Moon YJ, Kim SH, Kang H, Suk EH, Cho JH, Choi SS, et al. Endotracheal

intubation using semi-rigid optical stylet in simulated difficult airways of high grade modified Cormack and Lehane laryngeal views. Anesthesia and Pain Medicine. 2018;**13**:329-335. DOI: 10.17085/apm.2018.13.3.329

[42] Murashima K, Fukutome T. Effect of jaw-thrust manoeuvre on the laryngeal inlet. Anaesthesia. 1998;**53**:203-204

[43] Aoyama K, Takenaka I, Nagaoka E, Kadoya T. Jaw thrust maneuver for endotracheal intubation using a fiberoptic stylet. Anesthesia and Analgesia. 2000;**90**:1457-1458. DOI: 10.1097/00000539-200006000-00044

[44] Kleine-Brueggeney M, Greif R, Schoettker P, Savoldelli GL, Nabecker S, Theiler LG. Evaluation of six videolaryngoscopes in 720 patients with a simulated difficult airway: A multicentre randomized controlled trial. British Journal of Anaesthesia. 2016;**116**: 670-679. DOI: 10.1093/bja/aew058

[45] Suzuki K, Kusunoki S, Tanigawa K, Shime N. Comparison of three video laryngoscopes and direct laryngoscopy for emergency endotracheal intubation: a retrospective cohort study. BMJ Open. 2019;**9**(3):e024927. DOI: 10.1136/bmjopen-2018-024927

[46] Alvis BD, Hester D, Watson D, Higgins M, St JP. Randomized controlled trial comparing the McGrath MAC video laryngoscope with the king vision video laryngoscope in adult patients. Minerva Anestesiologica. 2016;**82**:30-35

[47] Mallick T, Verma A, Jaiswal S, Haldar M, Sheikh WR, Vishen A, et al. Comparison of the time to successful endotracheal intubation using the Macintosh laryngoscope or KingVision video laryngoscope in the emergency department: A prospective observational study. Turkish Journal of Emergency Medicine. 2020;**20**:22-27. DOI: 10.4103/2452-2473.276381

[48] Root CW, Mitchell OJL, Brown R, Evers CB, Boyle J, Griffin C, et al. Suction Assisted Laryngoscopy and Airway Decontamination (SALAD): A technique for improved emergency airway management. Resuscitation Plus. 2020;**1-2**:100005. DOI: 10.1016/j.resplu.2020.100005

[49] Ko S, Wong OF, Wong CHK, Ma HM, Lit CHA. A pilot study on using suction-assisted laryngoscopy airway decontamination techniques to assist endotracheal intubation by GlideScope® in a manikin simulating massive hematemesis. The Hong Kong Journal of Emergency Medicine. 2021;**28**:305-313. DOI: 10.1177/1024907919884206

[50] Paolini JB, Donati F, Drolet P. Review article: Video-laryngoscopy: Another tool for difficult intubation or a new paradigm in airway management? Canadian Journal of Anaesthesia. 2013; **60**:184-191. DOI: 10.1007/s12630-012-9859-5

[51] Matek J, Kolek F, Klementova O, Michalek P, Vymazal T. Optical devices in tracheal intubation-State of the art in 2020. Diagnostics (Basel). 2021;**11**(3): 575. DOI: 10.3390/diagnostics11030575

[52] Amir SH, Ali QE, Bansal S. A comparative evaluation of video stylet and flexible fibre-optic bronchoscope in the performance of intubation in adult patients. Indian Journal of Anaesthesia. 2017;**61**:321-325. DOI: 10.4103/ija.IJA_501_16

[53] Cho EA, Hwang SH, Lee SH, Ryu KH, Kim YH. Does glycopyrrolate premedication facilitate tracheal intubation with a rigid video-stylet?: A randomized controlled trial. Medicine

(Baltimore). 2018;**97**(32):e11834. DOI: 10.1097/MD.0000000000011834

[54] Chen IW, Chen JY, Lan KM, Hung KC. The use of Trachway for electromyographic (EMG) tube placement. Gland Surgery. 2018;7: 244-245. DOI: 10.21037/gs.2017.12.10

[55] Liu X, Zhang Y, Liu Z, Zhang Q, Wu W, Zheng Z, et al. Application of second-generation Shikani optical stylet in critically ill patients undergoing cerebral aneurysm embolization. The Journal of International Medical Research. 2019;**47**:1565-1572. DOI: 10.1177/0300060518822243

[56] Ma Y, Wang Y, Shi P, Cao X, Ge S. Ultrasound-guided versus Shikani optical stylet-aided tracheal intubation: A prospective randomized study. BMC Anesthesiology. 2020;**20**:221. DOI: 10.1186/s12871-020-01133-4

[57] Wahdan AS, El-Refai NAR, Omar SH, Abdel Moneem SA, Mohamed MM, Hussien MM. Endotracheal intubation in patients undergoing open abdominal surgery in the lateral position: A comparison between the intubating video stylet and fiberoptic intubating bronchoscopy. Korean Journal of Anesthesiology. 2021; **74**:234-241. DOI: 10.4097/kja.20384

[58] Godai K, Moriyama T, Kanmura Y. Comparison of the MultiViewScope stylet scope and the direct laryngoscope with the miller blade for the intubation in normal and difficult pediatric airways: A randomized, crossover, manikin study. PLoS One. 2020;**15**:e0237593. DOI: 10.1371/journal.pone.0237593

[59] Xu T, Li M, Ni C, Guo XY. Dexmedetomidine versus remifentanil for sedation during awake intubation using a Shikani optical stylet: A randomized, double-blinded, controlled trial. BMC Anesthesiology. 2016;**16**(1): 52. DOI: 10.1186/s12871-016-0219-9

[60] Costa F, Mattei A, Massimiliano C, Cataldo R, Agrò FE. The Clarus video system as a useful diagnostic tool. Anaesthesia. 2011;**66**:135-136. DOI: 10.1111/j.1365-2044.2010.06590.x

[61] Cooney DR, Cooney NL, Wallus H, Wojcik S. Performance of emergency physicians utilizing a video-assisted semi-rigid fiberoptic stylet for intubation of a difficult airway in a high-fidelity simulated patient: a pilot study. International Journal of Emergency Medicine. 2012;**5**(1):24. DOI: 10.1186/1865-1380-5-24

[62] Cooney DR, Beaudette C, Clemency BM, Tanski C, Wojcik S. Endotracheal intubation with a video-assisted semi-rigid fiberoptic stylet by prehospital providers. International Journal of Emergency Medicine. 2014;**7**: 45. DOI: 10.1186/s12245-014-0045-0

[63] Ong J, Lee CL, Lai HY, Lee Y, Chen TY, Shyr MH. A new video intubating device: Trachway intubating stylet. Anaesthesia. 2009;**64**(10):1145. DOI: 10.1111/j.1365-2044.2009.06092.x

[64] Ong J, Lee CL, Huang SJ, Shyr MH. Comparison between the Trachway video intubating stylet and Macintosh laryngoscope in four simulated difficult tracheal intubations: A manikin study. Tzu-Chi Medical Journal. 2016;**28**: 109-112. DOI: 10.1016/j.tcmj.2016.06.004

[65] Yang YL, Huang CH, Luk HN, Tsai PB. Adaptation to the plastic barrier sheet to facilitate intubation during the COVID-19 pandemic. Anesthesia and Analgesia. 2020;**131**:e97-e99. DOI: 10.1213/ANE.0000000000004923

[66] Luk HN, Yang YL, Huang CH, Su IM, Tsai PB. Application of plastic

sheet barrier and video intubating stylet to protect tracheal intubators during Coronavirus Disease 2019 pandemic: A Taiwan experience. Cell Transplant. 2021;**30**(Jan-Dec): 963689720987527. DOI: 10.1177/0963689720987527 Erratum in: Cell Transplant. 2021 Jan-Dec;30: 9636897211027078

[67] Tsai PB, Luk HN. Plastic sheet and video intubating stylet: A technical note. Asian Journal of Anesthesiology. 2021; **59**:117-121. DOI: 10.6859/aja.202109_59(3).0007

[68] Tsai PB, Luk HN. Sheet barrier and intubating stylet. Encyclopedia. 2021;**1**: 1058-1075. DOI: 10.3390/encyclopedia1040081

[69] Yang CP, Luk HN, Qu JZ, Shikani A. The use of a video-assisted intubating stylet technique in a critically ill and contagious COVID-19 patient. Healthcare (Basel). 2022;**10**(2):388. DOI: 10.3390/healthcare10020388

[70] Huang CH, Su IM, Jhuang BJ, Luk HN, Qu JZ, Shikani A. Video-assisted stylet intubation with a plastic sheet barrier, a safe and simple technique for tracheal intubation of COVID-19 patients. Healthcare. 2022; **10**:1105. DOI: 10.3390/healthcare10061105

[71] Weiss M, Schwarz U, Gerber AC. Difficult airway management: Comparison of the Bullard laryngoscope with the video-optical intubation stylet. Canadian Journal of Anaesthesia. 2000;**47**:280-284. DOI: 10.1007/BF03018927

[72] Aziz M, Metz S. Clinical evaluation of the Levitan optical stylet. Anaesthesia. 2011;**66**:579-581. DOI: 10.1111/j.1365-2044.2011.06708.x

[73] Lin YC, Cho AH, Lin JR, Chung YT. The Clarus video system (Trachway) and direct laryngoscope for endotracheal intubation with cricoid pressure in simulated rapid sequence induction intubation: A prospective randomized controlled trial. BMC Anesthesiology. 2019;**19**:33. DOI: 10.1186/s12871-019-0703-0

[74] Oh SH, Heo SK, Cheon SU, Ryu SA. The effects of backward, upward, rightward pressure maneuver for intubation using the Optiscope™: A retrospective study. Anesthesia and Pain Medicine (Seoul). 2021;**16**:391-397. DOI: 10.17085/apm.21026

[75] Moon YJ, Kim J, Seo DW, Kim JW, Jung HW, Suk EH, et al. Endotracheal intubation by inexperienced trainees using the Clarus video system: Learning curve and orodental trauma perspectives. Journal of Dental Anesthesia and Pain Medicine. 2015;**15**: 207-212. DOI: 10.17245/jdapm.2015.15.4.207

[76] Turkstra TP, Craen RA, Pelz DM, Gelb AW. Cervical spine motion: A fluoroscopic comparison during intubation with lighted stylet, GlideScope, and Macintosh laryngoscope. Anesthesia and Analgesia. 2005;**101**:910-915. DOI: 10.1213/01.ane.0000166975.38649.27

[77] Turkstra TP, Pelz DM, Shaikh AA, Craen RA. Cervical spine motion: A fluoroscopic comparison of Shikani optical stylet® vs Macintosh laryngoscope. Canadian Journal of Anaesthesia. 2007;**54**:441-447. DOI: 10.1007/BF03022029

[78] Kim JK, Kim JA, Kim CS, Ahn HJ, Yang MK, Choi SJ. Comparison of tracheal intubation with the airway scope or Clarus video system in patients with cervical collars. Anaesthesia. 2011;

66:694-698. DOI: 10.1111/j.1365-2044.2011.06762.x

[79] Seo H, Kim E, Son JD, Ji S, Min SW, Park HP. A prospective randomised study of a rigid video-stylet vs. conventional lightwand intubation in cervical spine-immobilised patients. Anaesthesia. 2016;**71**:1341-1346. DOI: 10.1111/anae.13606

[80] Nam K, Lee Y, Park HP, Chung J, Yoon HK, Kim TK. Cervical spine motion during tracheal intubation using an Optiscope versus the McGrath videolaryngoscope in patients with simulated cervical immobilization: A prospective randomized crossover study. Anesthesia and Analgesia. 2019;**129**: 1666-1672. DOI: 10.1213/ANE.0000000000003635

[81] Yoon HK, Lee HC, Park JB, Oh H, Park HP. McGrath MAC videolaryngoscope versus Optiscope video stylet for tracheal intubation in patients with manual inline cervical stabilization: A randomized trial. Anesthesia and Analgesia. 2020;**130**: 870-878. DOI: 10.1213/ANE.0000000000004442

[82] Chen YY, Lin JC, Tsai MJ, Cheng KY. Retromolar intubation with video intubating stylet in difficult airway: A randomized crossover manikin study. The American Journal of Emergency Medicine. 2022;**54**:212-220. DOI: 10.1016/j.ajem.2022.02.008

[83] Chan WH, Cheng CP, Chiu YL, Hsu YC, Hu MH, Huang GS. Two head positions for orotracheal intubation with the trachway videolight intubating stylet with manual in-line stabilization: A randomized controlled trial. Medicine (Baltimore). 2020;**99**:e19645. DOI: 10.1097/MD.0000000000019645

[84] Xu M, Li XX, Guo XY, Wang J. Shikani optical stylet versus macintosh laryngoscope for intubation in patients undergoing surgery for cervical spondylosis: A randomized controlled trial. Chinese Medical Journal. 2017;**130**: 297-302. DOI: 10.4103/0366-6999.198926

[85] Oh H, Kim H, Yoon HK, Lee HC, Park HP. No radiographic index predicts difficult intubation using the Optiscope™ in cervical spine surgery patients: A retrospective study. BMC Anesthesiology. 2020;**20**(1):47. DOI: 10.1186/s12871-020-00966-3

[86] Lin N, Li M, Shi S, Li TZ, Zhang BX. Shikani™ seeing optical stylet-aided tracheal intubation in patients with a large epiglottic cyst. Chinese Medical Journal. 2011;**124**:2795-2798

[87] Seo H, Lee G, Ha SI, Song JG. An awake double lumen endotracheal tube intubation using the Clarus video system in a patient with an epiglottic cyst: A case report. Korean Journal of Anesthesiology. 2014;**66**:157-159. DOI: 10.4097/kjae.2014.66.2.157

[88] Chen YT, Ho CN, Hung KC. Successful endotracheal intubation with Trachway after failed fiber-optic manipulations in a patient with retropharyngeal cervical chordoma. Tzu-Chi Medical Journal. 2017;**29**:174-176. DOI: 10.4103/tcmj.tcmj_63_17

[89] Cheng T, Wang LK, Wu HY, Yang XD, Zhang X, Jiao L. Shikani optical stylet for awake nasal intubation in patients undergoing head and neck surgery. The Laryngoscope. 2021;**131**: 319-325. DOI: 10.1002/lary.28763

[90] Yang M, Kim JA, Ahn HJ, Choi JW, Kim DK, Cho EA. Double-lumen tube tracheal intubation using a rigid video-stylet: A randomized controlled

comparison with the Macintosh laryngoscope. British Journal of Anaesthesia. 2013;**111**:990-995. DOI: 10.1093/bja/aet281

[91] Xu T, Li M, Guo XY. Comparison of Shikani optical stylet and Macintosh laryngoscope for double-lumen endotracheal tube intubation. Journal of Peking University (Health Sciences). 2015;**47**:853-858. DOI: 10.3969/j.issn.1671-167X.2015.05.024

[92] Xu T, Li M, Xu M, Guo X. Comparison of two shaping methods for double-lumen endotracheal tube intubation by Shikani optical stylet laryngoscope. Journal of Peking University (Health Sciences). 2016;**48**: 1038-1042. DOI: 10.3969/j.issn.1671-167X.2016.06.020

[93] Gaszynski T, Ewelina GE. The Clarus video system stylet for awake intubation in a very difficult urgent intubation. Anaesthesiology Intensive Therapy. 2013;**45**:153-154. DOI: 10.5603/AIT.2013.0032

[94] Tsay PJ, Yang CP, Luk HN, Qu JZ, Shikani A. Video-assisted intubating stylet technique for difficult intubation: A case series report. Healthcare (Basel). 2022;**10**(4):741. DOI: 10.3390/healthcare10040741

[95] Rosenstock CV, Thøgersen B, Afshari A, Christensen A, Eriksen C, Gätke MR. Awake fiberoptic or awake video laryngoscopic tracheal intubation in patients with anticipated difficult airway management: A randomized clinical trial. Anesthesiology. 2012;**116**: 1210-1216. DOI: 10.1097/ALN.0b013e318254d085

[96] Nowakowski M, Williams S, Gallant J, Ruel M, Robitaille A. Predictors of difficult intubation with the Bonfils rigid fiberscope. Anesthesia and Analgesia. 2016;**122**:1901-1906. DOI: 10.1213/ANE.0000000000001258

[97] Adnet F, Borron SW, Racine SX, Clemessy JL, Fournier JL, Plaisance P, et al. The intubation difficulty scale (IDS): Proposal and evaluation of a new score characterizing the complexity of endotracheal intubation. Anesthesiology. 1997;**87**:1290-1297. DOI: 10.1097/00000542-199712000-00005

[98] Harjai M, Alam S, Bhaskar P. Clinical relevance of Mallampati grading in predicting difficult intubation in the era of various new clinical predictors. Cureus. 2021;**13**(7):e16396. DOI: 10.7759/cureus.16396

[99] Brodsky JB, Lemmens HJ, Brock-Utne JG, Vierra M, Saidman LJ. Morbid obesity and tracheal intubation. Anesthesia and Analgesia. 2002;**94**: 732-736. DOI: 10.1097/00000539-200203000-00047

[100] Kristensen MS. Airway management and morbid obesity. European Journal of Anaesthesiology. 2010;**27**:923-927. DOI: 10.1097/EJA.0b013e32833d91aa

[101] Murphy C, Wong DT. Airway management and oxygenation in obese patients. Canadian Journal of Anaesthesia. 2013;**60**:929-945. DOI: 10.1007/s12630-013-9991-x

[102] Thota B, Jan KM, Oh MW, Moon TS. Airway management in patients with obesity. Saudi Journal of Anaesthesia. 2022;**16**:76-81. DOI: 10.4103/sja.sja_351_21

[103] Lavi R, Segal D, Ziser A. Predicting difficult airways using the intubation difficulty scale: A study comparing obese and non-obese patients. Journal of Clinical Anesthesia. 2009;**21**:264-267. DOI: 10.1016/j.jclinane.2008.08.021

[104] Siriussawakul A, Limpawattana P. A validation study of the intubation difficulty scale for obese patients. Journal of Clinical Anesthesia. 2016;**33**: 86-91. DOI: 10.1016/j.jclinane.2016.03.016

[105] Siriussawakul A, Maboonyanon P, Kueprakone S, Samankatiwat S, Komoltri C, Thanakiattiwibun C. Predictive performance of a multivariable difficult intubation model for obese patients. PLoS One. 2018; **13**(8):e0203142. DOI: 10.1371/journal.pone.0203142

[106] Neligan PJ, Porter S, Max B, Malhotra G, Greenblatt EP, Ochroch EA. Obstructive sleep apnea is not a risk factor for difficult intubation in morbidly obese patients. Anesthesia and Analgesia. 2009;**109**:1182-1186. DOI: 10.1213/ane.0b013e3181b12a0c

[107] Seo SH, Lee JG, Yu SB, Kim DS, Ryu SJ, Kim KH. Predictors of difficult intubation defined by the intubation difficulty scale (IDS): Predictive value of 7 airway assessment factors. Korean Journal of Anesthesiology. 2012;**63**: 491-497. DOI: 10.4097/kjae.2012.63.6.491

[108] Moon TS, Fox PE, Somasundaram A, Minhajuddin A, Gonzales MX, Pak TJ, et al. The influence of morbid obesity on difficult intubation and difficult mask ventilation. Journal of Anesthesia. 2019; **33**:96-102. DOI: 10.1007/s00540-018-2592-7

[109] Emik E, Gümüs-Özcan F, Demirgan S, Selcan A. Evaluation of the correlation between preoperative airway assessment tests, anthropometric measurements, and endotracheal intubation difficulty in obesity class III patients undergoing bariatric surgery. Medicine (Baltimore). 2021;**100**(36): e27188. DOI: 10.1097/MD.0000000000027188

[110] Gonzalez H, Minville V, Delanoue K, Mazerolles M, Concina D, Fourcade O. The importance of increased neck circumference to intubation difficulties in obese patients. Anesthesia and Analgesia. 2008;**106**: 1132-1136. DOI: 10.1213/ane.0b013e3181679659

[111] Kim WH, Ahn HJ, Lee CJ, Shin BS, Ko JS, Choi SJ, et al. Neck circumference to thyromental distance ratio: A new predictor of difficult intubation in obese patients. British Journal of Anaesthesia. 2011;**106**:743-748. DOI: 10.1093/bja/aer024

[112] Riad W, Vaez MN, Raveendran R, Tam AD, Quereshy FA, Chung F, et al. Neck circumference as a predictor of difficult intubation and difficult mask ventilation in morbidly obese patients: A prospective observational study. European Journal of Anaesthesiology. 2016;**33**:244-249. DOI: 10.1097/EJA.0000000000000324

[113] Özdilek A, Beyoglu CA, Erbabacan ŞE, Ekici B, Altındaş F, Vehid S, et al. Correlation of neck circumference with difficult mask ventilation and difficult laryngoscopy in morbidly obese patients: An observational study. Obesity Surgery. 2018;**28**:2860-2867. DOI: 10.1007/s11695-018-3263-3

[114] Wang T, Sun S, Huang S. The association of body mass index with difficult tracheal intubation management by direct laryngoscopy: A meta-analysis. BMC Anesthesiology. 2018;**18**(1):79. DOI: 10.1186/s12871-018-0534-4

[115] Keller C, Brimacombe J, Kleinsasser A, Brimacombe L. The laryngeal mask airway ProSeal™ as a

temporary ventilatory device in grossly and morbidly obese patients before laryngoscope-guided tracheal intubation. Anesthesia and Analgesia. 2002;**94**: 737-740. DOI: 10.1097/00000539-200203000-00048

[116] Wender R, Goldman AJ. Awake insertion of the fibreoptic intubating LMA CTrach™ in three morbidly obese patients with potentially difficult airways. Anaesthesia. 2007;**62**:948-951. DOI: 10.1111/j.1365-2044.2007.05127.x

[117] Arslan ZI, Özdamar D, Yildiz TS, Solak ZM, Toker K. Tracheal intubation in morbidly obese patients: A comparison of the intubating laryngeal mask airway™ and laryngeal mask airway CTrach™. Anaesthesia. 2012;**67**: 261-265. DOI: 10.1111/j.1365-2044.2011.06991.x

[118] Nicholson A, Cook TM, Smith AF, Lewis SR, Reed SS. Supraglottic airway devices versus tracheal intubation for airway management during general anaesthesia in obese patients. Cochrane Database of Systematic Reviews. 2013;**9**: CD010105. DOI: 10.1002/14651858.CD010105.pub2

[119] Nicholson A, Smith AF, Lewis SR, Cook TM. Tracheal intubation with a flexible intubation scope versus other intubation techniques for obese patients requiring general anaesthesia. Cochrane Database of Systematic Reviews. 2014;**1**: CD010320. DOI: 10.1002/14651858.CD010320.pub2

[120] Sun Y, Huang L, Xu L, Zhang M, Guo Y, Wang Y. The application of a SaCoVLM™ visual intubation laryngeal mask for the management of difficult airways in morbidly obese patients: Case report. Frontiers of Medicine (Lausanne). 2021;**8**:763103. DOI: 10.3389/fmed.2021.763103

[121] Yumul R, Elvir-Lazo OL, White PF, Sloninsky A, Kaplan M, Kariger R, et al. Comparison of three video laryngoscopy devices to direct laryngoscopy for intubating obese patients: A randomized controlled trial. Journal of Clinical Anesthesia. 2016;**31**:71-77. DOI: 10.1016/j.jclinane.2015.12.042

[122] Marrel J, Blanc C, Frascarolo P, Magnusson L. Videolaryngoscopy improves intubation condition in morbidly obese patients. European Journal of Anaesthesiology. 2007;**24**: 1045-1049. DOI: 10.1017/S0265021507000889

[123] Maassen R, Lee R, Hermans B, Marcus M, van Zundert A. A comparison of three videolaryngoscopes: The Macintosh laryngoscope blade reduces, but does not replace, routine stylet use for intubation in morbidly obese patients. Anesthesia and Analgesia. 2009;**109**:1560-1565. DOI: 10.1213/ANE.0b013e3181b7303a

[124] Andersen LH, Rovsing L, Olsen KS, GlideScope videolaryngoscope vs. Macintosh direct laryngoscope for intubation of morbidly obese patients: A randomized trial. Acta Anaesthesiologica Scandinavica. 2011;**55**:1090-1097. DOI: 10.1111/j.1399-6576.2011.02498.x

[125] Ydemann M, Rovsing L, Lindekaer AL, Olsen KS. Intubation of the morbidly obese patient: GlideScope® vs. Fastrach™. Acta Anaesthesiologica Scandinavica. 2012;**56**:755-761. DOI: 10.1111/j.1399-6576.2012.02693.x

[126] Moore AR, Schricker T, Court O. Awake videolaryngoscopy-assisted tracheal intubation of the morbidly obese. Anaesthesia. 2012;**67**:232-235. DOI: 10.1111/j.1365-2044.2011.06979.x

[127] Gaszyński T. Clinical experience with the C-mac videolaryngoscope in

morbidly obese patients. Anaesthesiology Intensive Therapy. 2014;**46**:14-16. DOI: 10.5603/AIT.2014.0003

[128] Arslan Zİ, Yörükoğlu HU. Tracheal intubation with the McGrath MAC X-blade videolaryngoscope in morbidly obese and nonobese patients. Turkish Journal of Medical Sciences. 2019;**49**: 1540-1546. DOI: 10.3906/sag-1901-169

[129] Brozek T, Bruthans J, Porizka M, Blaha J, Ulrichova J, Michalek P. A randomized comparison of non-channeled Glidescope™ titanium versus channeled KingVision™ videolaryngoscope for orotracheal intubation in obese patients with BMI > 35 kg m^{-2}. Diagnostics (Basel). 2020;**10**(12):1024. DOI: 10.3390/diagnostics10121024

[130] Ruetzler K, Rivas E, Cohen B, Mosteller L, Martin A, Keebler A, et al. McGrath video laryngoscope versus Macintosh direct laryngoscopy for intubation of morbidly obese patients: A randomized trial. Anesthesia and Analgesia. 2020;**131**:586-593. DOI: 10.1213/ANE.0000000000004747

[131] Bathory I, Granges JC, Frascarolo P, Magnusson L. Evaluation of the video intubation unit in morbid obese patients. Acta Anaesthesiologica Scandinavica. 2010;**54**:55-58. DOI: 10.1111/j.1399-6576.2009.02119.x

[132] Gaszynski T, Pietrzyk M, Szewczyk T, Gaszynska E. A comparison of performance of endotracheal intubation using the Levitan FPS optical stylet or Lary-flex videolaryngoscope in morbidly obese patients. Scientific World Journal. 2014;**2014**:207591. DOI: 10.1155/2014/207591

[133] Suppan L, Tramèr MR, Niquille M, Grosgurin O, Marti C. Alternative intubation techniques vs Macintosh laryngoscopy in patients with cervical spine immobilization: Systematic review and meta-analysis of randomized controlled trials. British Journal of Anaesthesia. 2016;**116**:27-36. DOI: 10.1093/bja/aev205

[134] Maharaj CH, Buckley E, Harte BH, Laffey JG. Endotracheal intubation in patients with cervical spine immobilization: A comparison of Macintosh and Airtraq laryngoscopes. Anesthesiology. 2007;**107**:53-59. DOI: 10.1097/01.anes.0000267529.71756.f0

[135] Robitaille A, Williams SR, Tremblay MH, Guilbert F, Thériault M, Drolet P. Cervical spine motion during tracheal intubation with manual in-line stabilization: Direct laryngoscopy versus GlideScope® videolaryngoscopy. Anesthesia and Analgesia. 2008;**106**: 935-941. DOI: 10.1213/ane.0b013e318161769e

[136] Malik MA, Maharaj CH, Harte BH, Laffey JG. Comparison of Macintosh, Truview EVO2®, Glidescope®, and Airwayscope® laryngoscope use in patients with cervical spine immobilization. British Journal of Anaesthesia. 2008;**101**:723-730. DOI: 10.1093/bja/aen231

[137] Enomoto Y, Asai T, Arai T, Kamishima K, Okuda Y. Pentax-AWS, a new videolaryngoscope, is more effective than the Macintosh laryngoscope for tracheal intubation in patients with restricted neck movements: A randomized comparative study. British Journal of Anaesthesia. 2008;**100**:544-548. DOI: 10.1093/bja/aen002

[138] Bathory I, Frascarolo P, Kern C, Schoettker P. Evaluation of the GlideScope® for tracheal intubation in

patients with cervical spine immobilisation by a semi-rigid collar. Anaesthesia. 2009;**64**:1337-1341. DOI: 10.1111/j.1365-2044.2009.06075.x

[139] Malik MA, Subramaniam R, Churasia S, Maharaj CH, Harte BH, Laffey JG. Tracheal intubation in patients with cervical spine immobilization: A comparison of the Airwayscope®, LMA CTrach®, and the Macintosh laryngoscopes. British Journal of Anaesthesia. 2009;**102**:654-661. DOI: 10.1093/bja/aep056

[140] Liu EH, Goy RW, Tan BH, Asai T. Tracheal intubation with videolaryngoscopes in patients with cervical spine immobilization: A randomized trial of the Airway Scope® and the GlideScope®. British Journal of Anaesthesia. 2009;**103**:446-451. DOI: 10.1093/bja/aep164

[141] Komatsu R, Kamata K, Sessler DI, Ozaki M. A comparison of the Airway Scope®and McCoy laryngoscope in patients with simulated restricted neck mobility. Anaesthesia. 2010;**65**:564-568. DOI: 10.1111/j.1365-2044.2010.06334.x

[142] McElwain J, Laffey JG. Comparison of the C-MAC®, Airtraq®, and Macintosh laryngoscopes in patients undergoing tracheal intubation with cervical spine immobilization. British Journal of Anaesthesia. 2011;**107**: 258-264. DOI: 10.1093/bja/aer099

[143] Kleine-Brueggeney M, Buttenberg M, Greif R, Nabecker S, Theiler L. Evaluation of three unchannelled videolaryngoscopes and the Macintosh laryngoscope in patients with a simulated difficult airway: A randomised, controlled trial. Anaesthesia. 2017;**72**:370-378. DOI: 10.1111/anae.13714

[144] Paik H, Park HP. Randomized crossover trial comparing cervical spine motion during tracheal intubation with a Macintosh laryngoscope versus a C-MAC D-blade videolaryngoscope in a simulated immobilized cervical spine. BMC Anesthesiology. 2020;**20**(1):201. DOI: 10.1186/s12871-020-01118-3

[145] Seo KH, Kim KM, John H, Jun JH, Han M, Kim S. Comparison of C-MAC D-blade videolaryngoscope and McCoy laryngoscope efficacy for nasotracheal intubation in simulated cervical spinal injury: a prospective randomized comparative study. BMC Anesthesiology. 2020;**20**(1):114. DOI: 10.1186/s12871-020-01021-x

[146] Yumul R, Elvir-Lazo OL, White PF, Durra O, Ternian A, Tamman R, et al. Comparison of the C-MAC video laryngoscope to a flexible fiberoptic scope for intubation with cervical spine immobilization. Journal of Clinical Anesthesia. 2016;**31**:46-52. DOI: 10.1016/j.jclinane.2015.12.045

[147] Kuo YM, Lai HY, Tan EC, Li YS, Chiang TY, Huang SS, et al. Cervical spine immobilization does not interfere with nasotracheal intubation performed using GlideScope videolaryngoscopy: A randomized equivalence trial. Scientific Reports. 2022;**12**(1):4041. DOI: 10.1038/s41598-022-08035-0

[148] Smereka J, Ladny JR, Naylor A, Ruetzler K, Szarpak L. C-MAC compared with direct laryngoscopy for intubation in patients with cervical spine immobilization: A manikin trial. The American Journal of Emergency Medicine. 2017;**35**:1142-1146. DOI: 10.1016/j.ajem.2017.03.030

[149] Park JW, An S, Park S, Nahm FS, Han SH, Kim JH. Comparison of a new video intubation stylet and McGrath® MAC video laryngoscope for intubation

in an airway manikin with normal airway and cervical spine immobilization scenarios by novice personnel: A randomized crossover study. BioMed Research International. 2021;**2021**: 4288367. DOI: 10.1155/2021/4288367

[150] Wang M, Ding R, Li Z, He M, Liu C. Comparison of intubation of Shikani optical stylet and Clarus video stylet in patients with cervical spine immobilization. The Journal of Practical Medicine. 2017;**24**:3933-3936

[151] Mahrous RSS, Ahmed AMM. The Shikani optical stylet as an alternative to awake fiberoptic intubation in patients at risk of secondary cervical spine injury: A randomized controlled trial. Journal of Neurosurgical Anesthesiology. 2018;**30**: 354-358. DOI: 10.1097/ANA.0000000000000454

[152] Cook TM, El-Boghdadly K, McGuire B, McNarry AF, Patel A, Higgs A. Consensus guidelines for managing the airway in patients with COVID-19: Guidelines from the Difficult Airway Society, the Association of Anaesthetists the Intensive Care Society, the Faculty of Intensive Care Medicine and the Royal College of Anaesthetists. Anaesthesia. 2020;**75**:785-799. DOI: 10.1111/anae.15054

[153] Brewster DJ, Chrimes N, Do TB, Fraser K, Groombridge CJ, Higgs A, et al. Consensus statement: Safe airway society principles of airway management and tracheal intubation specific to the COVID-19 adult patient group. The Medical Journal of Australia. 2020;**212**: 472-481. DOI: 10.5694/mja2.50598

[154] Yao W, Wang T, Jiang B, Gao F, Wang L, Zheng H, et al. Emergency tracheal intubation in 202 patients with COVID-19 in Wuhan, China: Lessons learnt and international expert recommendations. British Journal of Anaesthesia. 2020;**125**:e28-e37. DOI: 10.1016/j.bja.2020.03.026

[155] Chen X, Liu Y, Gong Y, Guo X, Zuo M, Li J, et al. Chinese Society of Anesthesiology, Chinese Association of Anesthesiologists. Perioperative management of patients infected with the novel coronavirus: Recommendation from the Joint Task Force of the Chinese Society of Anesthesiology and the Chinese Association of Anesthesiologists. Anesthesiology. 2020;**132**:1307-1316. DOI: 10.1097/ALN.0000000000003301

[156] Soh M, Hifumi T, Otani N, Maki K, Hayashi M, Miyazaki M, et al. Trends in endotracheal intubation for patients with COVID-19 by emergency physicians. Global Health & Medicine. 2022;**4**: 116-121. DOI: 10.35772/ghm.2021.01114

[157] Orser BA. Recommendations for endotracheal intubation of COVID-19 patients. Anesthesia and Analgesia. 2020;**130**:1109-1110. DOI: 10.1213/ANE.0000000000004803

[158] Saito T, Taguchi A, Asai T. Videolaryngoscopy for tracheal intubation in patients with COVID-19. British Journal of Anaesthesia. 2020;**125**: e284-e286. DOI: 10.1016/j.bja.2020.06.002

[159] Shrestha GS, Shrestha N, Lamsal R, Pradhan S, Shrestha A, Canelli R, et al. Emergency intubation in Covid-19. The New England Journal of Medicine. 2021; **384**(7):e20. DOI: 10.1056/NEJMvcm2007198

[160] Maslanka M, Smereka J, Czyzewski L, Ladny JR, Dabrowski M, Szarpak L. Vie scope® laryngoscope versus Macintosh laryngoscope with personal protective equipment during intubation of COVID-19 resuscitation patient. The American Journal of

Emergency Medicine. 2021;**46**:788-789. DOI: 10.1016/j.ajem.2020.08.085

[161] Grudzinski AL, Sun B, Zhang M, Crnic A, Djokhdem AH, Hanna M, et al. Airway recommendations for perioperative patients during the COVID-19 pandemic: A scoping review. Canadian Journal of Anaesthesia. 2022; **69**:644-657. DOI: 10.1007/s12630-022-02199-z

[162] Wong DJN, El-Boghdadly K, Owen R, Johnstone C, Neuman MD, Andruszkiewicz P, et al. Emergency airway management in patients with COVID-19: A prospective international multicenter cohort study. Anesthesiology. 2021;**135**:292-303. DOI: 10.1097/ALN.0000000000003791

[163] De Jong A, Pardo E, Rolle A, Bodin-Lario S, Pouzeratte Y, Jaber S. Airway management for COVID-19: A move towards universal videolaryngoscope? The Lancet Respiratory Medicine. 2020; **8**(6):555. DOI: 10.1016/S2213-2600(20)30221-6

[164] El-Orbany M, Connolly LA. Rapid sequence induction and intubation: Current controversy. Anesthesia and Analgesia. 2010;**110**:1318-1325. DOI: 10.1213/ANE.0b013e3181d5ae47

[165] Sajayan A, Wicker J, Ungureanu N, Mendonca C, Kimani PK. Current practice of rapid sequence induction of anaesthesia in the UK—A national survey. British Journal of Anaesthesia. 2016;**117**(Suppl. 1):i69-i74. DOI: 10.1093/bja/aew017

[166] Birenbaum A, Hajage D, Roche S, Ntouba A, Eurin M, Cuvillon P, et al. Effect of cricoid pressure compared with a sham procedure in the rapid sequence induction of anesthesia: The IRIS randomized clinical trial. JAMA Surgery. 2019;**154**:9-17. DOI: 10.1001/jamasurg.2018.3577

[167] Avery P, Morton S, Raitt J, Lossius HM, Lockey D. Rapid sequence induction: Where did the consensus go? Scandinavian Journal of Trauma, Resuscitation and Emergency Medicine. 2021;**29**(1):64. DOI: 10.1186/s13049-021-00883-5

[168] Sulser S, Ubmann D, Brueesch M, Goliasch G, Seifert B, Spahn DR, et al. The C-MAC videolaryngoscope compared with conventional laryngoscopy for rapid sequence intubation at the emergency department: study protocol. Scandinavian Journal of Trauma, Resuscitation and Emergency Medicine. 2015;**23**:38. DOI: 10.1186/s13049-015-0119-x

[169] Komasawa N, Kido H, Miyazaki Y, Tatsumi S, Minami T. Cricoid pressure impedes tracheal intubation with the Pentax-AWS Airwayscope®: A prospective randomized trial. British Journal of Anaesthesia. 2016;**116**:413-416. DOI: 10.1093/bja/aev438

[170] Asai T. Videolaryngoscopes: Do they have role during rapid-sequence induction of anaesthesia? British Journal of Anaesthesia. 2016;**116**:317-319. DOI: 10.1093/bja/aev544

[171] Kriege M, Lang P, Lang C, Pirlich N, Griemert EV, Heid F, et al. Anaesthesia protocol evaluation of the videolaryngoscopy with the McGrath MAC and direct laryngoscopy for tracheal intubation in 1000 patients undergoing rapid sequence induction: The randomised multicentre LARA trial study protocol. BMJ Open. 2021;**11**(10):e052977. DOI: 10.1136/bmjopen-2021-052977

[172] Purugganan RV, Jackson TA, Heir JS, Wang H, Cata JP. Video

laryngoscopy versus direct laryngoscopy for double-lumen endotracheal tube intubation: A retrospective analysis. Journal of Cardiothoracic and Vascular Anesthesia. 2012;**26**:845-848. DOI: 10.1053/j.jvca.2012.01.014

[173] Karczewska K, Bialka S, Smereka J, Cyran M, Nowak-Starz G, Chmielewski J, et al. Efficacy and safety of video-laryngoscopy versus direct laryngoscopy for double-lumen endotracheal intubation: A systematic review and meta-analysis. Journal of Clinical Medicine. 2021;**10**(23):5524. DOI: 10.3390/jcm10235524

[174] Yoo JY, Park SY, Kim JY, Kim M, Haam SJ, Kim DH. Comparison of the McGrath videolaryngoscope and the Macintosh laryngoscope for double lumen endobronchial tube intubation in patients with manual in-line stabilization: A randomized controlled trial. Medicine (Baltimore). 2018;**97**(10): e0081. DOI: 10.1097/MD.0000000000010081

[175] Risse J, Schubert AK, Wiesmann T, Huelshoff A, Stay D, Zentgraf M, et al. Videolaryngoscopy versus direct laryngoscopy for double-lumen endotracheal tube intubation in thoracic surgery—A randomised controlled clinical trial. BMC Anesthesiol. 2020; **20**(1):150. DOI: 10.1186/s12871-020-01067-x

[176] Wasem S, Lazarus M, Hain J, Festl J, Kranke P, Roewer N, et al. Comparison of the Airtraq and the Macintosh laryngoscope for double-lumen tube intubation: A randomised clinical trial. European Journal of Anaesthesiology. 2013;**30**:180-186. DOI: 10.1097/EJA.0b013e32835fe574

[177] Yao WL, Wan L, Xu H, Qian W, Wang XR, Tian YK, et al. A comparison of the McGrath® series 5 videolaryngoscope and Macintosh laryngoscope for double-lumen tracheal tube placement in patients with a good glottic view at direct laryngoscopy. Anaesthesia. 2015;**70**:810-817. DOI: 10.1111/anae.13040

[178] El-Tahan MR, Khidr AM, Gaarour IS, Alshadwi SA, Alghamdi TM, Al'ghamdi A. A comparison of 3 videolaryngoscopes for double-lumen tube intubation in humans by users with mixed experience: A randomized controlled study. Journal of Cardiothoracic and Vascular Anesthesia. 2018;**32**:277-286. DOI: 10.1053/j.jvca.2017.08.009

[179] Kim YS, Song J, Lim BG, Lee IO, Won YJ. Different classes of videoscopes and direct laryngoscopes for double-lumen tube intubation in thoracic surgery: A systematic review and network meta-analysis. PLoS One. 2020; **15**(8):e0238060. DOI: 10.1371/journal.pone.0238060

[180] Yi J, Gong Y, Quan X, Huang Y. Comparison of the Airtraq laryngoscope and the GlideScope for double-lumen tube intubation in patients with predicted normal airways: A prospective randomized trial. BMC Anesthesiology. 2015;**15**:58. DOI: 10.1186/s12871-015-0037-5

[181] Hsu HT, Chou SH, Chen CL, Tseng KY, Kuo YW, Chen MK, et al. Left endobronchial intubation with a double-lumen tube using direct laryngoscopy or the Trachway® video stylet. Anaesthesia. 2013;**68**:851-855. DOI: 10.1111/anae.12340

[182] Kim YR, Jun BH, Kim JA. The use of the Clarus video system for double-lumen endobronchial tube intubation in a patient with a difficult airway. Korean Journal of Anesthesiology. 2013;**65**: 85-86. DOI: 10.4097/kjae.2013.65.1.85

[183] Hossfeld B, Frey K, Doerges V, Lampl L, Helm M. Improvement in glottic visualisation by using the C-MAC PM video laryngoscope as a first-line device for out-of-hospital emergency tracheal intubation: An observational study. European Journal of Anaesthesiology. 2015;**32**:425-431. DOI: 10.1097/EJA.00000000000 00249

[184] De Jong A, Molinari N, Conseil M, Coisel Y, Pouzeratte Y, Belafia F, et al. Video laryngoscopy versus direct laryngoscopy for orotracheal intubation in the intensive care unit: A systematic review and meta-analysis. Intensive Care Medicine. 2014;**40**:629-639. DOI: 10.1007/s00134-014-3236-5

[185] Park SO, Kim JW, Na JH, Lee KH, Lee KR, Hong DY, et al. Video laryngoscopy improves the first-attempt success in endotracheal intubation during cardiopulmonary resuscitation among novice physicians. Resuscitation. 2015;**89**:188-194. DOI: 10.1016/j.resuscitation.2014.12.010

[186] Sakles JC, Mosier JM, Patanwala AE, Dicken JM, Kalin L, Javedani PP. The C-MAC® video laryngoscope is superior to the direct laryngoscope for the rescue of failed first-attempt intubations in the emergency department. The Journal of Emergency Medicine 2015;48: 280-286. DOI: 10.1016/j.jemermed.2014.10.007

[187] Kim JW, Park SO, Lee KR, Hong DY, Baek KJ, Lee YH, et al. Video laryngoscopy vs. direct laryngoscopy: Which should be chosen for endotracheal intubation during cardiopulmonary resuscitation? A prospective randomized controlled study of experienced intubators. Resuscitation. 2016;**105**:196-202. DOI: 10.1016/j.resuscitation.2016.04.003

[188] Hypes CD, Stolz U, Sakles JC, Joshi RR, Natt B, Malo J, et al. Video laryngoscopy improves odds of first-attempt success at intubation in the intensive care unit. A propensity-matched analysis. Annals of the American Thoracic Society. 2016;**13**: 382-390. DOI: 10.1513/AnnalsATS.201508-505OC

[189] Risse J, Volberg C, Kratz T, Plöger B, Jerrentrup A, Pabst D, et al. Comparison of videolaryngoscopy and direct laryngoscopy by German paramedics during out-of-hospital cardiopulmonary resuscitation; an observational prospective study. BMC Emergency Medicine. 2020;**20**(1):22. DOI: 10.1186/s12873-020-00316-z

[190] Hossfeld B, Thierbach S, Allgoewer A, Gaessler H, Helm M. First pass success of tracheal intubation using the C-MAC PM videolaryngoscope as first-line device in prehospital cardiac arrest compared with other emergencies: An observational study. European Journal of Anaesthesiology. 2021;**38**: 806-812. DOI: 10.1097/EJA.0000000000001286

[191] Nouruzi-Sedeh P, Schumann M, Groeben H. Laryngoscopy via Macintosh blade versus GlideScope: Success rate and time for endotracheal intubation in untrained medical personnel. Anesthesiology. 2009;**110**:32-37. DOI: 10.1097/ALN.0b013e318190b6a7

[192] Kory P, Guevarra K, Mathew JP, Hegde A, Mayo PH. The impact of video laryngoscopy use during urgent endotracheal intubation in the critically ill. Anesthesia and Analgesia. 2013;**117**: 144-149. DOI: 10.1213/ANE.0b013e3182917f2a

[193] Silverberg MJ, Li N, Acquah SO, Kory PD. Comparison of video laryngoscopy versus direct laryngoscopy

during urgent endotracheal intubation: A randomized controlled trial. Critical Care Medicine. 2015;**43**:636-641. DOI: 10.1097/CCM.0000000000000751

[194] Lee DH, Han M, An JY, Jung JY, Koh Y, Lim CM, et al. Video laryngoscopy versus direct laryngoscopy for tracheal intubation during in-hospital cardiopulmonary resuscitation. Resuscitation. 2015;**89**:195-199. DOI: 10.1016/j.resuscitation.2014.11.030

[195] Bhattacharjee S, Maitra S, Baidya DK. A comparison between video laryngoscopy and direct laryngoscopy for endotracheal intubation in the emergency department: A meta-analysis of randomized controlled trials. Journal of Clinical Anesthesia. 2018;**47**:21-26. DOI: 10.1016/j.jclinane.2018.03.006

[196] Russell TM, Hormis A, Rotherham NHS Foundation Trust. Should the Glidescope video laryngoscope be used first line for all oral intubations or only in those with a difficult airway? A review of current literature. Journal of Perioperative Practice. 2018;**28**:322-333. DOI: 10.1177/1750458918788985

[197] Keresztes D, Mérei Á, Rozanovic M, Nagy E, Kovács-Ábrahám Z, Oláh J, et al. Comparison of VividTrac, King Vision and Macintosh laryngoscopes in normal and difficult airways during simulated cardiopulmonary resuscitation among novices. PLoS One. 2021;**16**(11): e0260140. DOI: 10.1371/journal.pone.0260140

[198] Griesdale DE, Liu D, McKinney J, Choi PT. Glidescope® video-laryngoscopy versus direct laryngoscopy for endotracheal intubation: A systematic review and meta-analysis. Canadian Journal of Anaesthesia. 2012; **59**:41-52. DOI: 10.1007/s12630-011-9620-5

[199] Huang HB, Peng JM, Xu B, Liu GY, Du B. Video laryngoscopy for endotracheal intubation of critically ill adults: A systemic review and meta-analysis. Chest. 2017;**152**:510-517. DOI: 10.1016/j.chest.2017.06.012

[200] Szarpak L, Madziala A, Czekajlo M, Smereka J, Kaserer A, Dabrowski M, et al. Comparison of the UEScope videolaryngoscope with the Macintosh laryngoscope during simulated cardiopulmonary resuscitation: A randomized, cross-over, multi-center manikin study. Medicine (Baltimore). 2018;**97**(36):e12085. DOI: 10.1097/MD.0000000000012085

[201] Arulkumaran N, Lowe J, Ions R, Mendoza M, Bennett V, Dunser MW. Videolaryngoscopy versus direct laryngoscopy for emergency orotracheal intubation outside the operating room: A systematic review and meta-analysis. British Journal of Anaesthesia. 2018;**120**: 712-724. DOI: 10.1016/j.bja.2017.12.041

[202] Ba X. A meta-analysis on the effectiveness of video laryngoscopy versus laryngoscopy for emergency orotracheal intubation. Journal of Healthcare Engineering. 2022;**2022**: 1474298. DOI: 10.1155/2022/1474298

[203] Sulser S, Ubmann D, Schlaepfer M, Brueesch M, Goliasch G, Seifert B, et al. C-MAC videolaryngoscope compared with direct laryngoscopy for rapid sequence intubation in an emergency department: A randomised clinical trial. European Journal of Anaesthesiology. 2016;**33**:943-948. DOI: 10.1097/EJA.0000000000000525

[204] Schuerner P, Grande B, Piegeler T, Schlaepfer M, Saager L, Hutcherson MT, et al. Hands-off time for endotracheal intubation during CPR is not altered by the use of the C-MAC video-laryngoscope compared to conventional

direct laryngoscopy. A randomized crossover manikin study. PLoS One. 2016;**11**(5):e0155997. DOI: 10.1371/journal.pone.0155997

[205] Jiang J, Kang N, Li B, Wu AS, Xue FS. Comparison of adverse events between video and direct laryngoscopes for tracheal intubations in emergency department and ICU patients-a systematic review and meta-analysis. Scandinavian Journal of Trauma, Resuscitation and Emergency Medicine. 2020;**28**(1):10. DOI: 10.1186/s13049-020-0702-7

[206] Wu MY, Yiang GT, Ke JY, Chen CS, Lin PC, Chen YL. Role of Trachway versus conventional modes of intubation in difficult airway management in COVID-19 setups. Emergency Medicine International. 2021;**2021**:6614523. DOI: 10.1155/2021/6614523

[207] Ray DC, Billington C, Kearns PK, Kirkbride R, Mackintosh K, Reeve CS, et al. A comparison of McGrath and Macintosh laryngoscopes in novice users: A manikin study. Anaesthesia. 2009;**64**: 1207-1210. DOI: 10.1111/j.1365-2044.2009.06061.x

[208] Reus E, Grundmann U, Liening K, Wrobel M. Parker flex-it intubation stylet versus a 90-degree curved stylet during intubation with the McGrath videolaryngoscope performed by novices: A manikin study with 5 airway scenarios. Journal of Clinical Anesthesia. 2013;**25**:624-628. DOI: 10.1016/j.jclinane.2013.07.001

[209] Kotera A, Irie H, Iwashita S, Taniguchi J, Kasaoka S, Kinoshita Y. Comparison of the conventional Macintosh laryngoscope, the Pentax Airwayscope, and the McGrath MAC video laryngoscope under restricted cervical motion: A manikin study. Acute Medicine & Surgery. 2014;**2**:138-142. DOI: 10.1002/ams2.88

[210] Choi JW, Kim JA, Jung HJ, Kim WH. Tracheal intubation with a McGrath® series 5 video laryngoscope by novice personnel in a cervical-immobilized manikin. The Journal of Emergency Medicine. 2016;**50**:61-66. DOI: 10.1016/j.jemermed.2015.06.079

[211] Madziala M, Smereka J, Dabrowski M, Leung S, Ruetzler K, Szarpak L. A comparison of McGrath MAC® and standard direct laryngoscopy in simulated immobilized cervical spine pediatric intubation: A manikin study. European Journal of Pediatrics. 2017;**176**: 779-786. DOI: 10.1007/s00431-017-2909-9

[212] Yi IK, Kwak HJ, Lee KC, Lee JH, Min SK, Kim JY, et al. Pentax, and Macintosh laryngoscope in normal and cervical immobilized manikin by novices: A randomized crossover trial. European Journal of Medical Research. 2020;**25**(1):35. DOI: 10.1186/s40001-020-00435-0

[213] Ghotbaldinian E, Dehdari N, Åkeson J. Maintenance of basic endotracheal intubation skills with direct or video-assisted laryngoscopy: A randomized crossover follow-up study in inexperienced operators. AEM Education and Training. 2021;**5**(4): e10655. DOI: 10.1002/aet2.10655

[214] Gadek L, Szarpak L, Konge L, Dabrowski M, Telecka-Gadek D, Maslanka M, et al. Direct vs. video-laryngoscopy for intubation by paramedics of simulated COVID-19 patients under cardiopulmonary resuscitation: A randomized crossover trial. Journal of Clinical Medicine. 2021; **10**(24):5740. DOI: 10.3390/jcm10245740

[215] Johnston LC, Auerbach M, Kappus L, Emerson B, Zigmont J, Sudikoff SN. Utilization of exploration-based learning and video-assisted

learning to teach GlideScope videolaryngoscopy. Teaching and Learning in Medicine. 2014;**26**:285-291. DOI: 10.1080/10401334.2014.910462

[216] Sakles JC, Mosier J, Patanwala AE, Dicken J. Learning curves for direct laryngoscopy and GlideScope® video laryngoscopy in an emergency medicine residency. The Western Journal of Emergency Medicine. 2014;**15**:930-937. DOI: 10.5811/westjem.2014.9.23691

[217] Pius J, Ioanidis K, Noppens RR. Use of the novel C-MAC video stylet in a case of predicted difficult intubation: A case report. A&A Practice. 2019;**13**:88-90. DOI: 10.1213/XAA.0000000000000998

[218] Pius J, Noppens RR. Learning curve and performance in simulated difficult airway for the novel C-MAC® video-stylet and C-MAC® Macintosh video laryngoscope: A prospective randomized manikin trial. PLoS One. 2020;**15**(11): e0242154. DOI: 10.1371/journal.pone.0242154

[219] Tseng KY, Chau SW, Su MP, Shih CK, Lu IC, Cheng KI. A comparison of Trachway intubating stylet and airway scope for tracheal intubation by novice operators: A manikin study. The Kaohsiung Journal of Medical Sciences. 2012;**28**:448-451. DOI: 10.1016/j.kjms.2012.02.016

[220] Hung KC, Tan PH, Lin VC, Wang HK, Chen HS. A comparison of the Trachway intubating stylet and the Macintosh laryngoscope in tracheal intubation: A manikin study. Journal of Anesthesia. 2013;**27**:205-210. DOI: 10.1007/s00540-012-1491-6

[221] Kriege M, Alflen C, Strauß H, Ott T, Noppens RR. Usage of a semi-rigid intubation endoscope is not superior to a video laryngoscope. A prospective, randomised, controlled trial comparing the SensaScope vs. the McGrath series 5 in surgical patients. Trends in Anaesthesia and Critical Care. 2018;**18**: 23-28. DOI: 10.1016/j.tacc.2018.01.003

[222] Wang HY, Lin C, Chen CC, Teng WN, Chen KH, Lo MT, et al. Improvement in vocal-cord visualization with Trachway video intubating stylet using direct oxygen flow and effective analysis of the fraction of inspired oxygen: A bench study. Journal of Clinical Monitoring and Computing. 4 March 2022. DOI: 10.1007/s10877-022-00818-0 [Online ahead of print]

[223] Sharma D, Kim LJ, Ghodke B. Successful airway management with combined use of Glidescope® videolaryngoscope and fiberoptic bronchoscope in a patient with Cowden syndrome. Anesthesiology. 2010;**113**: 253-255. DOI: 10.1097/ALN.0b013e3181dfd334

[224] Gu J, Xu K, Ning J, Yi B, Lu K. GlideScope-assisted fiberoptic bronchoscope intubation in a patient with severe rheumatoid arthritis. Acta Anaesthesiologica Taiwanica. 2014;**52**: 85-87. DOI: 10.1016/j.aat.2014.04.002

[225] Ara T, Mori G, Adachi E, Asai T, Okuda Y. Combined use of the GlideScope and fiberoptic bronchoscope for tracheal intubation in a patient with difficult airway. Masui. 2014;**63**:647-649 PMID: 24979855

[226] Liew GHC, Wong TGL, Lu A, Kothandan H. Combined use of the Glidescope and flexible fibrescope as a rescue technique in a difficult airway. Proceedings of Singapore Healthcare. 2015;**June**:117-120. DOI: 10.1177/201010581502400208

[227] Loh PS, Ng KWS. Combining glidescope and fiber-optic for intubation in oral maxillofacial surgery. Journal of

Anaesthesiology Clinical Pharmacology. 2017;**33**:254-255. DOI: 10.4103/0970-9185.209738

[228] Chung MY, Park B, Seo J, Kim CJ. Successful airway management with combined use of McGrath® MAC video laryngoscope and fiberoptic bronchoscope in a severe obese patient with huge goiter-a case report. Korean Journal of Anesthesiology. 2018;**71**:232-236. DOI: 10.4097/kja.d.18.27203

[229] Sanfilippo F, Sgalambro F, Chiaramonte G, Santonocito C, Burgio G, Arcadipane A. Use of a combined laryngo-bronchoscopy approach in difficult airways management: A pilot simulation study. Turkish Journal of Anaesthesiology & Reanimation. 2019;**47**:464-470. DOI: 10.5152/TJAR.2019.99234

[230] Kim SM, Kim HJ. Successful advancement of endotracheal tube with combined fiberoptic bronchoscopy and videolaryngoscopy in a patient with a huge goiter. SAGE Open Medical Case Reports. 2020;**8**:2050313X20923232. DOI: 10.1177/2050313X20923232

[231] Kim JY, Yeom JY, Youn SJ, Lee JE, Oh JY, Byun SH. Fiberoptic-guided nerve integrity monitoring tube intubation assisted by video-laryngoscope with external laryngeal manipulation in a patient with anteriorly displaced larynx due to huge goiter with retropharyngeal involvement: A case report. Medicine (Baltimore). 2022;**101**(10):e29041. DOI: 10.1097/MD.0000000000029041

[232] Maybauer MO, Maier S, Thierbach AR. An unexpected difficult intubation. Bonfils rigid fiberscope. Anaesthesist. 2005;**54**:35-40. DOI: 10.1007/s00101-004-0772-3

[233] Liao X, Xue FS, Cheng Y, Li RP. Rescue intubation by combined use of video laryngoscopy and Bonfils fiberscope in patients with difficult airway. Saudi Medical Journal. 2013;**34**:970-971. PMID: 24043013

[234] Lim H, Cha YB, Ryu KH, Lee SH, Cho EA. Comparison of two different shapes of stylets for intubation with the McGrath MAC® video laryngoscope: A randomized controlled trial. The Journal of International Medical Research. 2020;**48**(10):300060520962951. DOI: 10.1177/0300060520962951

[235] Young CF, Vadivelu N. Does the use of a laryngoscope facilitate orotracheal intubation with a Shikani optical stylet? British Journal of Anaesthesia. 2007;**99**:302-303. DOI: 10.1093/bja/aem196

[236] Kim SH, Woo SJ, Kim JH. A comparison of Bonfils intubation fiberscopy and fiberoptic bronchoscopy in difficult airways assisted with direct laryngoscopy. Korean Journal of Anesthesiology. 2010;**58**:249-255. DOI: 10.4097/kjae.2010.58.3.249

[237] Kovacs G, Law JA, McCrossin C, Vu M, Leblanc D, Gao J. A comparison of a fiberoptic stylet and a bougie as adjuncts to direct laryngoscopy in a manikin-simulated difficult airway. Annals of Emergency Medicine. 2007;**50**:676-685. DOI: 10.1016/j.annemergmed.2007.05.022

[238] Chang PY, Hu PY, Lin YC, Chen HY, Chiang FY, Wu CW, et al. Trachway video intubating stylet allows for optimization of electromyographic endotracheal tube placement for monitored thyroidectomy. Gland Surgery. 2017;**6**:464-468. DOI: 10.21037/gs.2017.08.08

[239] Aziz MF, Dillman D, Fu R, Brambrink AM. Comparative effectiveness of the C-MAC video laryngoscope versus direct laryngoscopy in the setting of the predicted difficult airway. Anesthesiology. 2012;**116**: 629-636. DOI: 10.1097/ALN.0b013e318246ea34

Chapter 5

Difficult Airway in Obstetric Patients

Glenardi Glenardi

Abstract

Although the use of general anesthesia in the obstetric population has decreased substantially, it remains the most appropriate choice in certain cases. While the use of general anesthesia is essential, maternal deaths associated with general anesthesia continue. Difficult airway remains the leading cause. Maternal mortality due to airway difficulty during general anesthesia is approximately four times higher than in general population. The incidence of failed tracheal intubation in obstetrics has remained unchanged over the past 40 years. The significant anatomic and physiologic changes of pregnancy, which are exacerbated during labor, explain the increased difficulty in airway management in obstetric patients. The presence of anesthesia staff with adequate knowledge of maternal airway management is vital to minimize the incidence of failed intubation in the parturient.

Keywords: obstetric anesthesia, difficult airway, airway management, failed intubation, general anesthesia

1. Introduction

Although the use of general anesthesia (GA) has been largely replaced by neuraxial anesthesia, there are certain clinical situations in which the administration of GA is most appropriate [1, 2]. GA is frequently preferred in emergent cases (e.g., fetal bradycardia, massive hemorrhage, maternal coagulopathy, uterine rupture, maternal trauma) as it has a rapid onset and allows for airway ventilation and hemodynamic control [2, 3]. Airway-related complications remain a leading cause of anesthesia-related maternal mortality [2–7], with approximately 2.3 per 100,000 GAs versus 1 per 180,000 GAs in the general population. Although advanced airway devices (e.g., supraglottic airways, flexible bronchoscopes, and video laryngoscopy) have been increasingly available for difficult airway management, the incidence of failed tracheal intubation in obstetrics cases has remained unchanged over the past 40 years. A 2015 systematic review reported that the incidence of failed intubation for all obstetric procedures was 1 in 390 [8]. The rate of failed obstetric intubation is approximately eight times higher compared with non-obstetric procedures [9]. Significant anatomic and physiological changes of pregnancy have been considered to explain the increased difficulty in obstetric airway management [2–4]. Several suggestions have been proposed to reduce the difficulty of maternal airway management [10, 11].

2. Anatomic and physiologic risk factors for airway complications in obstetric patients

Pregnancy results in multiple anatomic and physiological changes, which impact airway management. While respiratory changes have the most significant effect, there are also gastroesophageal and other pregnancy-induced changes that increase the risk for difficult airway management.

2.1 Respiratory changes

Increases in the renin-aldosterone system result from augmented estrogen and progesterone production during normal pregnancy cause a physiological fluid retention [11, 12]. In the respiratory tract, this may lead to narrowing of the airway, increasing risk for airway obstruction during ventilation, poor laryngoscopic views, and difficulty with tracheal intubation [2, 3]. Although airway changes develop gradually from first to third trimester of pregnancy, even more drastic changes may be observed at delivery and during labor. Studies have shown an increase in the Mallampati score and a decrease in upper airway volume on acoustic reflectometry during labor, presumably due to increasing soft tissue edema [13, 14]. Rather than relying solely on prelabor assessment, it is necessary to reevaluate the airway immediately prior to induction of general anesthesia as the airway edema may be exacerbated during the second stage of labor following fluid resuscitation [13, 15, 16]. Capillary engorgement of airway mucosal lining in pregnant women can increase the risk for bleeding during manipulation of the upper airway, especially in the nasal cavity [2, 3]. Consequently, many practitioners are reluctant to perform a nasal intubation as it has higher risk for epistaxis during pregnancy [2]. However, a 2011 review from Arendt et al. suggests that nasal intubation is acceptable with proper preparation of the nasal mucosa using topical vasoconstrictors, and the intubation is performed by the fiberoptic nasotracheal intubation technique [17]. However, an individual assessment is required prior to this procedure, as topical vasoconstrictors may have an impact on maternal hemodynamic and uteroplacental perfusion [2].

Physical derangements of pregnancy increase the risk of maternal and fetal hypoxemia during induction of anesthesia and subsequent airway manipulation. As the gravid uterus expands toward diaphragm, functional residual capacity (FRC) decreases by approximately 20–30% at term. This reduction comprises a 25% reduction in expiratory reserve volume (ERV) and a 15% reduction in residual volume (RV) [2, 18, 19]. The reduction is more prominent during a supine position. Although FRC decreases significantly, the closing capacity (CC) remains unchanged in pregnancy, resulting in a reduced FRC/CC ratio. Consequently, more rapid closure of the small airways may occur, increasing the risk of atelectasis [2, 3, 20]. In addition to the upward movement of the diaphragm, there are also other diaphragm changes that occur as pregnancy advances: lengthening of muscle fibers, an increase in the zone of apposition, and an increase in the radius of curvature of the diaphragm [21–23]. These changes contribute to an increase in ribcage dimension and concurrent tidal volume increase of up to 45% at term [21, 22, 24]. Along with the increased respiratory rate that is observed during pregnancy, an approximately 48% increase is observed in minute ventilation during the first trimester. Due to increased minute ventilation, maternal $PaCO_2$ decreases and arterial pH increases causing a mild respiratory alkalosis (typically 7.42–7.44) [3]. As the pregnancy progresses, oxygen consumption also increases significantly [2, 3, 25]. An approximately 60% increase in oxygen demand is observed during pregnancy as the fetus grows. Consequently, pregnant women are more susceptible to developing hypoxemia during the induction of GA [25].

2.2 Gastroesophageal changes

During pregnancy, the esophagus, stomach, and pylorus are displaced cephalad by the enlarging uterus, decreasing the competence of the lower esophageal sphincter (LES). Elevated levels of progesterone and estrogen during pregnancy further reduce LES tone [2, 3, 18]. In addition, gastrin secretion increases during pregnancy, leading to increased gastric hydrogen ion production, and thereby increasing gastric pressure. This increase in gastric pressure, plus the incompetence of the LES, increases risks of regurgitation, aspiration, and the development of esophagitis and acid pneumonitis [2, 3]. Although the increased risk of regurgitation and aspiration does not necessarily result in difficult laryngoscopy and intubation, it has been reported to cause death during general anesthesia [26].

Gastric emptying time is not prolonged during pregnancy compared with the nonpregnant women [27]. However, it begins to prolong with the onset of labor, due to pain, anxiety, and the administration of analgesics. It also further contributes to the increased risk of regurgitation and aspiration in pregnant women. Therefore, it is prudent to consider all pregnant women at increased risk for pulmonary aspiration during labor [2, 3].

2.3 Other changes

Most women gain between 10 and 15 kg during pregnancy due to increase in uterine size, fetal mass, fat deposition, blood, and interstitial fluid volume [18]. This may increase the risk of difficult airway management, as high BMI is associated with more difficult mask ventilation, laryngoscopy, and tracheal intubation, especially in short stature women. Moreover, a more rapid oxygen desaturation during the induction of GA is also associated with people with higher BMI. In addition to pregnancy-related weight gain, breast enlargement during pregnancy is also associated with more difficult laryngoscopy. Therefore, optimizing intubation position is necessary to facilitate correct placement of the laryngoscope blade [2, 3].

3. Airway assessment

Preanesthetic assessment of the airway should be performed, when possible, to detect the potential of difficulty airway [2, 3, 28, 29]. Preanesthetic assessment should consist of history taking and physical [3]. Any history of difficult airway management is vital in preanesthetic airway assessment [30]. Presence of pathological conditions associated with a difficult airway should also be noted, including snoring, which may make mask ventilation more difficult [31, 32]. A complete physical examination should always be performed to detect the physical characteristics associated with difficult airway. There are five specific components of the airway exam that should be evaluated: overall inspection of the face and neck, oropharyngeal and dental anatomy, neck anatomy and range of motion, mandibular protrusion ability, and submandibular space [3].

The overall inspection of face and neck is necessary to detect any pathological states involving the face or neck, such as massive face deformities, facial burns, retrognathia, tumor involving the face or neck, thick or short neck, or large goiter [3]. In the setting of pregnancy and trauma, the presence of a cervical collar has been shown to interfere with mask ventilation and direct laryngoscopy [33].

There are two important components in oropharyngeal and dental examination that should be evaluated: maximum voluntary mouth opening and Mallampati score [3]. Measurement of maximum mouth opening is achieved by measuring the inter-incisor distance when the patient voluntarily opens the mouth as wide as possible [3, 34, 35]. Inter-incisor distance of less than 3 cm, or 2 fingerbreadths, is associated with difficult intubation [34]. Some studies even suggest that a distance of less than 4–4.5 cm can increase the risk of a difficult airway [35]. In 1983, Mallampati et al. described a clinical sign to determine the difficulty of direct laryngoscopy and tracheal intubation, based on the size and position of the tongue relative to the pharyngeal size. To assess the Mallampati classification, the patient should be in an upright sitting position with the head in a neutral position, the mouth wide open, and the tongue protruding as far as possible without phonation. Higher scores on the Mallampati classification indicate more difficult laryngoscopy and tracheal intubation, because the tongue is large enough to obscure oropharyngeal view. The original version of Mallampati classification consisted of a three-point scale [36]. However, Samsoon and Young further modified the Mallampati classification into a four-point scale (see **Table 1**) [9].

The dental condition of the patient has also been shown to affect airway management [34]. To prevent trauma and tooth aspiration, it is recommended to extract very loose teeth prior to laryngoscopy. Although the edentulous patient is almost always associated with easy tracheal intubation, face mask ventilation is often difficult [37].

A thick neck (neck circumference greater than 43 cm) has been shown to increase the risk of difficult tracheal intubation [33, 38]. In addition, neck mobility is also essential in airway examination as it is necessary to have an ideal neck position when doing laryngoscopy and intubation. The ideal intubating position is achieved by the extension of the atlantooccipital joint, in what is called the sniffing position, with the alignment of the oral, pharyngeal, and laryngeal axes. Normal atlantooccipital joint extension should be greater than 35° [39, 40]. Moreover, the sternomental distance can also be used to quantitatively assess neck mobility. The sternomental distance is the distance between the chin point and the sternal notch, measured when the head is in extension and the mouth is closed. Distance less than 12.5 cm has shown to increase the risk of difficult intubation [41]. Overall neck range of motion also can be used to predict the risk of difficult intubation. The assessment is performed by measuring the angle between forehead and neck when fully flexed and extended. An angle of less than 80° is associated with difficult intubation [42].

The mandibular protrusion test has been shown to have strong predictive value in determining a difficult laryngoscopy. It is performed by instructing the patient to

Class	Definition
Class 1	When the soft palate, fauces, uvula, and faucial pillars are visible
Class 2	When the soft palate, fauces, and the uvula are visible
Grade 3	When the soft palate and the base of uvula are visible
Grade 4	When only the soft palate is visible

Table 1.
Modified Mallampati classification [9].

Class	Definition
Class 1	The lower incisor is able to bite the upper lip above the vermilion border
Class 2	The lower incisor is able to bite the upper lip below the vermilion border
Class 3	The lower incisor is not able to bite the upper lip

Table 2.
The upper lip bite test classification [44].

extend the mandible as far as possible and then assessing the location of the mandibular teeth in comparison to the maxillary teeth. When the mandibular teeth can extend beyond the maxillary teeth, it is predictive of easy laryngoscopy [43]. Similar to mandibular protrusion test, the upper lip bite test (ULBT) is also shown to have predictive value in determining the likelihood of difficult airway, with higher specificity than the Mallampati classification. In the ULBT, the patient is instructed to bite their upper lip. The ability of biting the upper lip is then classified into three classes (see **Table 2**). The higher the class, the more difficult it is to laryngoscope and intubate [44, 45].

Evaluation of submandibular space is essential in determining the risk of difficult laryngoscopy and intubation. During direct laryngoscopy, the blade of the laryngoscope displaces the tongue into the submandibular space. A small submandibular space will cause inadequate visualization of the glottis. The submandibular space can be estimated by measuring the thyromental distance. It is measured from the lower border of the mentum to the thyroid cartilage notch. A distance of less than 6.5 cm or 3 fingerbreadths suggests an increased risk of difficult intubation [46, 47].

In pregnant women, a recent study found that the modified Mallampati test was shown to have better predictive value compared with ULBT, thyromental distance, and sternomental distance. In addition, this study also showed that the best cutoff point for the thyroid distance was 5 cm and for the sternomental distance was 15 cm. However, combining these various tests suggested to have a better diagnostic accuracy [48]. Moreover, several new modalities such as bedside endoscopy, point-of-care ultrasonography (POCUS), virtual laryngoscopy/bronchoscopy, or three-dimensional printing can be used to further evaluate the risk of airway difficulty, especially in patients with complex airway pathology [28].

4. Management

Management of the obstetric difficult airway requires adequate preoperative preparation, a throughout intraoperative plan, and multiple back-up plans. All practitioners should be familiar with the algorithms for anticipated and unanticipated difficult airway in OB.

4.1 Preoperative preparation

Preoperative preparation should consist of obtaining informed consent, assessing the airway, determining fasting policy, and administering premedication [49]. Prior to obtaining informed consent, the anesthesiologist must provide the patient with comprehensive information regarding the risks and benefits of the GA procedure in the obstetric population. It should also include possible airway management that may be undertaken to address possible airway difficulties during the procedure. Even if airway examination indicates no risk of difficult airway, it risk of unanticipated or unrecognized airway issues and complications is not eliminated. Therefore, the anesthesiologist should always have a management plan for unanticipated airway difficulties even before the general anesthesia is initiated [2, 50].

In addition to increased gastric pressure during pregnancy, prolonged gastric emptying during labor has also been shown to increase the risk of regurgitation and aspiration in laboring women. Therefore, it has been historically recommended to avoid ingesting solid food and clear fluid 6 and before 2 h, respectively, before the operative procedure [51, 52]. As the incidence of maternal death caused by aspiration decreases, more studies are suggesting liberal nil per oral (NPO) guidelines, allowing ingestion of isotonic fluids and light diet during labor [53]. Moreover, several premedication drugs are also used as aspiration prophylaxis. The purpose of these drug is to reduce pH and the amount of gastric volume. The aspiration prophylactic drugs include histamine-2 receptor antagonists (e.g., ranitidine), proton-pump inhibitors (e.g., omeprazole, lansoprazole), nonparticulate antacid (e.g., sodium citrate), or promotility drugs (e.g., metoclopramide) [49, 50, 54, 55]. The use of histamine-2 receptor antagonists with or without a promotility drug is the most common regimen for aspiration prophylaxis in the obstetric patient. Ranitidine and metoclopramide should be administered at least 30 min before induction [56, 57]. In emergent situation, a dose of sodium citrate 30 mL may also be used within 30 min of surgery [56, 58, 59].

In addition to patient preparation, the anesthesiologist should also have a discussion with the team whether to proceed with the procedure or wake the patient in the event of failed tracheal intubation [2, 49]. The Obstetric Anesthetists' Association and Difficult Airway Society (OAA/DAS) provides guidelines for this decision (see **Figure 1**).

Table 1 – proceed with surgery?

	Factors to consider	WAKE	⟵	⟶	PROCEED
Before induction	Maternal condition	• No compromise	• Mild acute compromise	• Haemorrhage responsive to resuscitation	• Hypovolaemia requiring corrective surgery • Critical cardiac or respiratory compromise, cardiac arrest
	Fetal condition	• No compromise	• Compromise corrected with intrauterine resuscitation, pH < 7.2 but > 7.15	• Continuing fetal heart rate abnormality despite intrauterine resuscitation, pH < 7.15	• Sustained bradycardia • Fetal haemorrhage • Suspected uterine rupture
	Anaesthetist	• Novice	• Junior trainee	• Senior trainee	• Consultant/specialist
	Obesity	• Supermorbid	• Morbid	• Obese	• Normal
	Surgical factors	• Complex surgery or major haemorrhage anticipated	• Multiple uterine scars • Some surgical difficulties expected	• Single uterine scar	• No risk factors
	Aspiration risk	• Recent food	• No recent food • In labour • Opioids given • Antacids not given	• No recent food • In labour • Opioids not given • Antacids given	• Fasted • Not in labour • Antacids given
	Alternative anaesthesia • regional • securing airway awake	• No anticipated difficulty	• Predicted difficulty	• Relatively contraindicated	• Absolutely contraindicated or has failed • Surgery started
After failed intubation	Airway device/ ventilation	• Difficult facemask ventilation • Front-of-neck	• Adequate facemask ventilation	• First generation supraglottic airway device	• Second generation supraglottic airway device
	Airway hazards	• Laryngeal oedema • Stridor	• Bleeding • Trauma	• Secretions	• None evident

Figure 1.
Factors to consider in the decision to procced with surgery or wake the patient following failed tracheal intubation. Reproduced from Mushambi et al. [49], with permission from obstetric Anesthetists' association/difficult airway society.

4.2 Rapid sequence induction and intubation

To minimize the risk of aspiration, rapid sequence induction and intubation (RSI) has become the standard induction technique in obstetric general anesthesia [2, 60–62]. The goal of RSI is to minimize the length of time between loss of consciousness and the establishment of optimal intubating condition. In the traditional RSI technique, after achieving ideal patient position, preoxygenation, and application of cricoid pressure, the administration of an intravenous induction agent is then rapidly followed by administration of an intravenous neuromuscular blocking agent; the trachea is intubated without attempts at positive-pressure ventilation (PPV) [3, 60]. The goal of avoiding PPV is to prevent gastric insufflation, as this may increase the risk of regurgitation [63]. However, OAA/DAS recommends considering the use of facemask ventilation, as the risk of regurgitation is low with correct application of cricoid pressure. Therefore, the steps in performing RSI in obstetric patient are: (1) proper patient positioning; (2) preoxygenation; (3) application of cricoid pressure; (4) administration of induction agent and neuromuscular blocking agent; (5) face mask ventilation; (6) tracheal intubation [49].

In obstetric procedures, propofol is the typical induction agent, barring hemodynamic or respiratory concerns. After the administration of induction agent, neuromuscular blocking drugs (NMDs) are then administered intravenously to facilitate optimal intubating condition. Succinylcholine or suxamethonium has historically been the most commonly used NMD for RSI in obstetric patients because of its rapid onset and short duration, allowing resumption of spontaneous ventilation in the event of failed intubation [2, 3, 64]. The optimal dose of succinylcholine is 1–1.5 mg/kg [3, 65–67]. Although the level of plasma pseudocholinesterase decreases during pregnancy, studies show that the duration of action of succinylcholine in pregnant women remains unchanged [68]. Since the advent of sugammadex, a fast-acting reversal agent specifically for rocuronium or vecuronium, nondepolarizing NMDs (e.g., rocuronium, vecuronium) can also be used in RSI technique as the alternative to succinylcholine [64, 69, 70]. The optimal dose of rocuronium is 1–1.2 mg/kg, and vecuronium is 0.3 mg/kg [71–75]. Sugammadex (16 mg/kg) can rapidly reverse the effects of rocuronium or vecuronium to prevent the prolong duration of action. Therefore, it can achieve the same clinical effects as succinylcholine without risk of hyperkalemia, bradycardia, myalgia, increased intragastric pressure, and increased intracranial pressure [71–76].

In contrast to standard RSI, modified RSI with low-pressure ventilation (<12 cm H_2O) with correct application of cricoid pressure, is recommended in RSI for obstetric patients. Ventilation is carried out using a facemask with a maximum inflation pressure of 20 cm H_2O. The goal of PPV is to delay the onset of hypoxemia and increase the likelihood of successful facemask ventilation in the event of difficult or failed tracheal intubation [77, 78].

In pregnant women without risk of difficult airway, direct laryngoscopy using a Macintosh blade is preferred [2, 3, 79]. However, in patients at risk of difficult airway (e.g., obese) and those who fail tracheal intubation, practitioners should use a video laryngoscope to provide a better view of the glottis and thereby increase the chances of success [80–90]. Since all obstetric patients are at a higher risk for a difficult airway, video laryngoscope should always be available in all obstetric general anesthetics [49, 79]. If the view of the glottis is not optimal during the first laryngoscopy, the anesthesiologist may reduce or remove cricoid pressure and reposition the head and neck [91, 92]. Due to capillary engorgement and edema of the mucosal lining of the airway in pregnant women, the risk for airway obstruction and bleeding during upper airway manipulation is higher than in the general population [13, 14]. Therefore, a small endotracheal tube (e.g., size 6.5 or 7.0) is recommended to minimize the risk of trauma and increase the success rate in pregnant women. To minimize the risk of pulmonary aspiration, a cuffed endotracheal tube is used. In addition, endotracheal tube introducer (e.g., flexible stylet, bougie) can be used to improve the success rate of tracheal intubation [2, 49].

4.3 Management of the unanticipated difficult airway

Anesthesiologists must be prepared to manage difficult airway situations. Algorithms for the unanticipated difficult airway in the parturient have been developed by national and international organizations.

If intubation fails on the first attempt, a second attempt should be made by a more experienced anesthetist using alternative equipment as appropriate. Ventilation via facemask is recommended if there is a delay in the second attempt. During the second attempt at intubation, cricoid pressure should not be applied (see **Figure 2**) [49]. In addition, a second attempt at intubation should not be continued if there is a Cormack-Lehane grade 3b or 4 view at laryngoscopy to prevent airway trauma and loss of airway control [49, 93–95]. In case of two unsuccessful intubations, the anesthesiologist should declare a failed intubation and proceed to the failed intubation algorithm according to the OAA/DAS guideline (see **Figure 2**). However, in the presence of experienced anesthetist, this guideline also allows for a maximum of three attempts at intubation before declaring a failed intubation [49, 96].

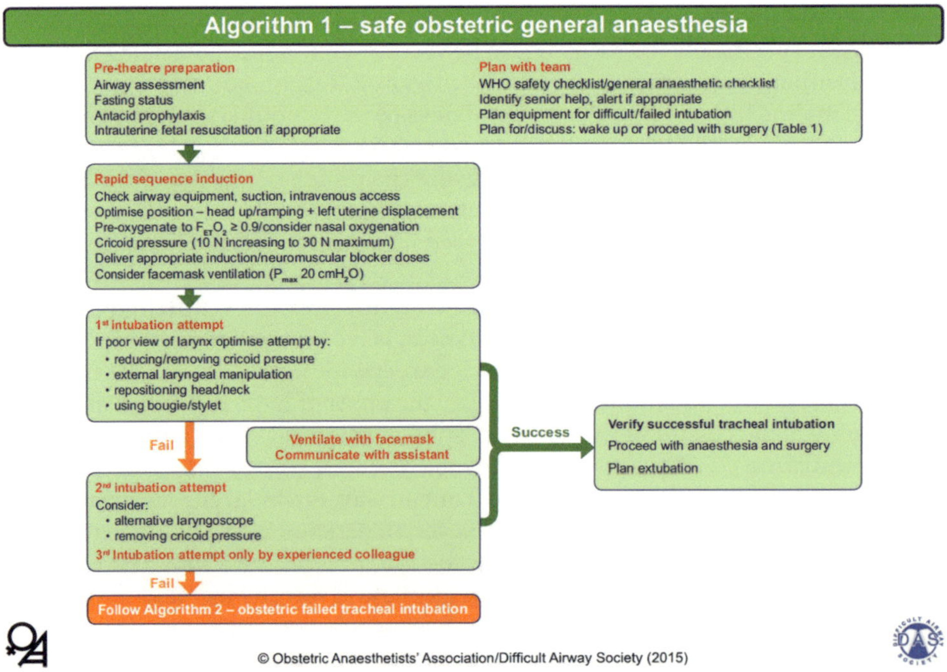

Figure 2.
Safe obstetric general anesthesia. Reproduced from Mushambi et al. [49], with permission from obstetric Anesthetists' association/difficult airway society.

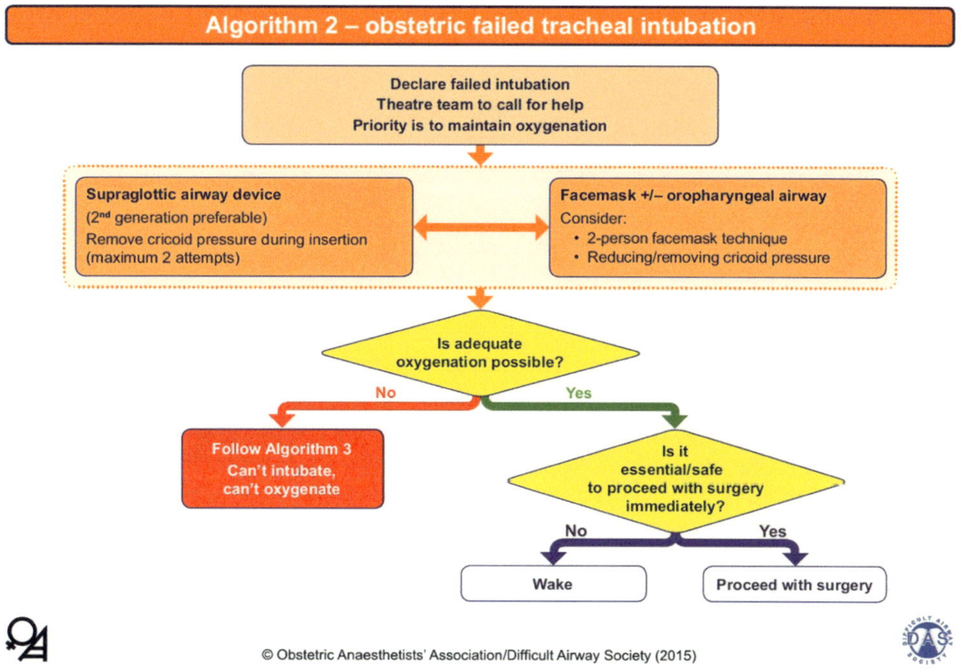

Figure 3.
Management of failed tracheal intubation in obstetrics. Reproduced from Mushambi et al. [49], with permission from obstetric Anesthetists' association/difficult airway society.

If a failed intubation has been declared, airway management consists of three steps including (1) calling for help, (2) maintaining adequate oxygenation, (3) determining whether proceed or wake the patient (see **Figure 3**) [49]. A more experienced anesthesiologist should be called immediately to help in airway management [2, 3, 28, 29, 49]. To maintain adequate oxygenation, ventilation can be performed through a facemask or supraglottic airway device. When performing facemask ventilation, it is recommended to use the two-person (four-handed) technique and to reduce or release the cricoid pressure [28, 29, 49]. If facemask ventilation is found to be difficult or inadequate, a supraglottic airway device should be inserted immediately before the effects of the induction agent and NMD wear off [49]. The second-generation supraglottic airway device is recommended as it has an additional esophageal drainage port and oropharyngeal cuff to reduce the risk of pulmonary aspiration [28, 29, 49]. During the insertion of supraglottic airway device, cricoid pressure should be temporarily removed. Only two attempts at supraglottic device insertion should be performed in order to prevent bleeding or further airway trauma. Once the adequate oxygenation has been established, the anesthetist and team should determine whether to proceed with surgery or wake the patient. The final decision should be based on consideration of several factors that have been evaluated preoperatively (see **Figure 1**) [49] However, the presence of airway hazards and the degree of difficulty in airway management remain major factors in decision-making because maternal safety is a top priority for the anesthesiologist. If there is no evidence of a difficult airway or a life-threatening condition for the mother, the safest strategy is to awaken the mother. If the mother is in immediate jeopardy and no other anesthetic technique is feasible, anesthetist should consider proceeding with surgery. On the other hand, if the mother is stable with a life-threatening condition of the fetus, it is advisable to consider waking the mother. Despite the controversial decision, the risks of an unsecured airway and the increased risk of aspiration are considered to outweigh the benefits of proceeding with surgery [2, 49]. This is a difficult decision, and evidence does support both sides. Several studies have shown that continuing surgery with a well-functioning supraglottic airway device following failed tracheal intubation is considered as safe and is also recommended [29, 97].

In the setting of a failed intubation, if the decision is made to wake the patient, the anesthesiologist must maintain adequate oxygenation and prevent pulmonary aspiration by applying cricoid pressure and changing the patient position to head-up or left-lateral position. In addition, the anesthesiologist should also assess for the possibility of persistent paralysis and laryngeal spasm. If there is persistent paralysis, sugammadex can be used to reverse the effects of rocuronium. To anticipate the occurrence of laryngeal spasm and "can't intubate, can't oxygenate" (CICO) situations, the anesthesiologist must also prepare the appropriate equipment, drugs, and personnel. Following waking, the obstetrician should review the urgency of delivery, and anesthetist should consider the safest alternative anesthetic option for the patient. Options for anesthetic technique include (1) regional anesthesia or (2) general anesthesia preceded by awake intubation or tracheostomy [2, 49]. If regional anesthesia is selected, anesthetist should prepare for a backup plan in case high or failed block happened. If general anesthesia is selected, awake intubation using video laryngoscope or flexible bronchoscope with topical anesthesia is recommended [49, 98, 99]. However, in the event of extreme difficulty or failure of tracheal intubation via upper airway, tracheostomy should be performed immediately [49].

If the decision to proceed with surgery has been made in the setting of failed intubation, anesthesiologist should consider the following issues: (1) maintenance

Table 2 – management after failed tracheal intubation

Wake

- Maintain oxygenation
- Maintain cricoid pressure if not impeding ventilation
- Either maintain head-up position or turn left lateral recumbent
- If rocuronium used, reverse with sugammadex
- Assess neuromuscular blockade and manage awareness if paralysis is prolonged
- Anticipate laryngospasm/can't intubate, can't oxygenate

After waking

- Review urgency of surgery with obstetric team
- Intrauterine fetal resuscitation as appropriate
- For repeat anaesthesia, manage with two anaesthetists
- Anaesthetic options:
  - Regional anaesthesia preferably inserted in lateral position
  - Secure airway awake before repeat general anaesthesia

Proceed with surgery

- Maintain anaesthesia
- Maintain ventilation - consider merits of:
  - controlled or spontaneous ventilation
  - paralysis with rocuronium if sugammadex available
- Anticipate laryngospasm/can't intubate, can't oxygenate
- Minimise aspiration risk:
  - maintain cricoid pressure until delivery (if not impeding ventilation)
  - after delivery maintain vigilance and reapply cricoid pressure if signs of regurgitation
  - empty stomach with gastric drain tube if using second-generation supraglottic airway device
  - minimise fundal pressure
  - administer H_2 receptor blocker i.v. if not already given
- Senior obstetrician to operate
- Inform neonatal team about failed intubation
- Consider total intravenous anaesthesia

Figure 4.
Management after failed tracheal intubation in obstetrics. Reproduced from Mushambi et al. [49], with permission from obstetric Anesthetists' association/difficult airway society.

of anesthesia, (2) selection of airway device, (3) maintenance of ventilation, (4) strategy to prevent pulmonary aspiration. To maintain adequate anesthesia, a non-irritant volatile agent such as sevoflurane is commonly used. In the event of uterine atony after delivery, total intravenous anesthesia with propofol may be considered as it has no effect on uterine muscle tone [49]. If a failed intubation has been declared, the anesthesiologist must choose whether to proceed with only a supraglottic airway device or to perform additional tracheal intubation attempts [29]. Although the use of supraglottic airway device is not advisable in elective surgery, its use in caesarian delivery has found to be effective and safe [29, 49, 97]. Again, a second-generation of supraglottic airway device is recommended. If the anesthetist decides to proceed with additional attempt at tracheal intubation, it should be noted that only one attempt by an experienced anesthesiologist with a planned intubation technique should be allowed [29]. The intubation technique must overcome the anatomical constraints that led to the earlier failure. Although the selection of intubation technique depends on anesthesiologist's clinical judgment, it is recommended to use flexible bronchoscope-guided intubation to avoid airway trauma and esophageal intubation [29, 100]. If tracheal intubation fails to be performed safely, a definitive airway with tracheostomy is required [29, 49]. Although controlled ventilation is used in the vast majority of failed intubation cases in the United Kingdom, a case-by-case consideration should be exercised before deciding whether to use spontaneous or controlled ventilation [49, 79]. In addition, to prevent pulmonary aspiration during the procedure, cricoid pressure should be applied until after delivery (**Figures 4** and **5**) [49].

Following failed tracheal intubation, persistent failure to ventilate using facemask and supraglottic airway device leads to a "can't intubate, can't oxygenate" (CICO)

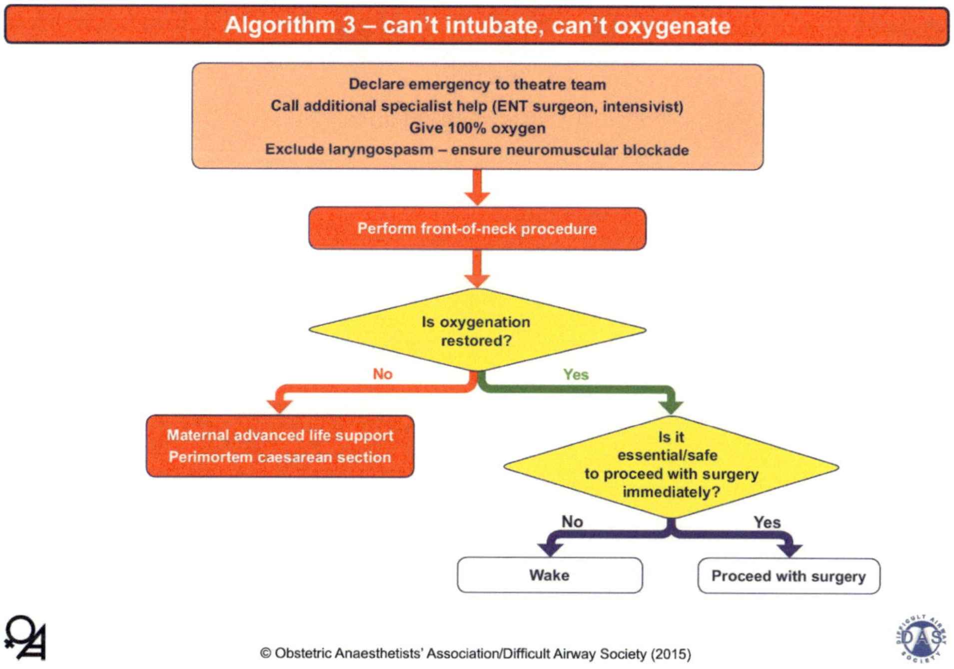

Figure 5.
Management of "can't intubate, can't oxygenate" (CICO) in obstetrics. Reproduced from Mushambi et al. [49], with permission from obstetric Anesthetists' association/difficult airway society.

situation. The CICO situation may be caused by poor chest wall compliance and laryngeal spasm, which can be managed with NMDs [28, 29, 49]. Therefore, once a CICO situation has been identified, apart from calling an ear, nose, and throat surgeon and/or intensivist, it is imperative to rule out laryngeal spasm as the cause of CICO. The reason is to prevent invasive airway management when it can be managed with only NMD [29, 49]. If the succinylcholine has been administered during induction, then a combination of rocuronium and sugammadex is preferred [29, 49, 50]. When laryngospasm has been ruled out as the cause of CICO, front-of-neck procedure should proceed without delay. A front-of-neck procedure refers to procedure to securing airway access via front of the neck by either tracheotomy or cricothyrotomy [29]. Prior to front-of-neck procedure, patient should inhale 100% oxygen via a facemask or supraglottic airway device while waiting for the neuromuscular blockade to be confirmed or established [49]. Once the neuromuscular blockade has been established, front-of-neck procedure can be performed immediately. If an experienced surgeon is present, tracheotomy may be performed to provide definitive airway access [29, 101, 102]. However, cricothyrotomy may be more preferred in emergency setting [29, 50]. If adequate oxygenation is not achieved, a cardiac arrest protocol should be instituted, and undelivered fetus at >20 weeks' gestation age should be delivered via cesarean section immediately [49, 103].

4.4 Management of the anticipated difficult airway

Anticipated difficult airway is defined as a clinical situation in which a trained anesthesiologist has anticipated difficulty in providing ventilation using facemask or a supraglottic airway, laryngoscopy, tracheal intubation, extubation, or invasive airway [104]. In pregnant women with an anticipated difficult airway, neuraxial anesthesia is more preferred compared with general anesthesia as it does not require any airway manipulation. However, anesthetist should always have backup plan for securing the airway in case high or failed block happened. If pregnant women with anticipated difficult airway must undergo general anesthesia, the safest option is to perform awake tracheal intubation [2].

4.5 Extubation of the trachea

Pulmonary aspiration is the one of the most common adverse events at the end of anesthesia, especially during the extubation [6, 105]. In obstetric patients, awake extubation is recommended. The position during extubation is also important to prevent regurgitation [49]. Recent study suggests a head-up position because it aids the patency of airway, respiratory function, and access to the airway [106].

5. Conclusion

Although the use of general anesthesia (GA) has been largely replaced by neuraxial anesthesia, in certain obstetric situations, GA is preferred. Advantages include rapid control of the airway and ventilation, improved hemodynamic control, and speed of onset. While maternal mortality associated with GA has decreased substantially, deaths from difficult airway in GA are still reported and are higher in obstetric patients compared with the general population. One of the leading causes of airway-related death during obstetric GA is difficult and failed intubation. The significant anatomic and physiologic changes of pregnancy have been considered to explain the increased difficulty in airway management in obstetric patients. Airway mucosal edema, capillary swelling, decreased functional residual capacity, and increased oxygen consumption during pregnancy have been shown to cause difficult airway in obstetric patients. In addition, gastroesophageal changes during pregnancy, such as decreased lower esophageal sphincter muscle competence, increased gastric pressure, and prolonged gastric emptying, are associated with an increased risk of pulmonary aspiration in pregnant women. These changes may be further exacerbated during labor; therefore, some modifications are needed in the obstetric airway management. These modifications include using certain specific equipment, administering additional premedication, performing additional procedures, and using different airway management algorithms. Therefore, it is necessary to have adequate knowledge regarding the management of difficult airways in obstetrics to prevent future airway-related mortality and morbidity of mothers and neonates.

Conflict of interest

The authors declare no conflict of interest.

Abbreviations

GA	general anesthesia
FRC	functional residual capacity
ERV	expiratory reserve volume
RV	residual volume
CC	closing capacity
ULBT	upper lip bite test
POCUS	point-of-care ultrasonography
CAFG	Canadian Airway Focus Group
CICO	cannot intubate, cannot oxygenate
CVCO	cannot ventilate, cannot oxygenate
OAA/DAS	Obstetric Anesthetists' Association and Difficult Airway Society
RSI	rapid sequence induction and intubation
PPV	positive-pressure ventilation
FETO2	end-tidal oxygen fraction
NMDs	neuromuscular blocking drugs
eFONA	emergency front of neck access

Author details

Glenardi Glenardi
Atma Jaya Catholic University of Indonesia, Jakarta, Indonesia

*Address all correspondence to: glenardihalim@gmail.com

References

[1] Traynor AJ, Aragon M, Ghosh D, Choi RS, Dingmann C, Vu Tran Z, et al. Obstetric anesthesia workforce survey: A 30-year update. Anesthesia & Analgesia. 2016;**122**(6):1939-1946

[2] Tawfik MM, Tolba MA. Chestnut's obstetric Anesthesia: Principles and practice, 6th ed. Anesthesia & Analgesia. 2019;**129**(5):p170

[3] Gropper MA, Miller RD, Eriksson LI, Fleisher LA, Wiener-Kronish JP, Cohen NH, et al. Miller's Anesthesia, 2-Volume Set E-book. Amsterdam: Elsevier Health Sciences; 2019

[4] Delgado C, Ring L, Mushambi MC. General anaesthesia in obstetrics. BJA education. 2020;**20**(6):201

[5] Knight M, Nair M, Tuffnell D, Kenyon S, Shakespeare J, Brocklehurst P, et al. Saving Lives, Improving Mothers' Care: Surveillance of Maternal Deaths in the UK 2012-14 and Lessons Learned to Inform Maternity Care from the UK and Ireland Confidential Enquiries into Maternal Deaths and Morbidity 2009-14. Oxuniprint. Oxford: University of Oxford; 2016

[6] Knight M, Kenyon S, Brocklehurst P, Neilson J, Shakespeare J, Kurinczuk JJ. Saving Lives, Improving mothers' Care-Lessons Learned to Inform Future Maternity Care from the UK and Ireland Confidential Enquiries into Maternal Deaths and Morbidity 2009-2012. National Perinatal Epidemiology Unit: University of Oxford; 2014

[7] Creanga AA, Syverson C, Seed K, Callaghan WM. Pregnancy-related mortality in the United States, 2011-2013. Obstetrics and gynecology. 2017;**130**(2):366

[8] Kinsella SM, Winton AL, Mushambi MC, Ramaswamy K, Swales H, Quinn AC, et al. Failed tracheal intubation during obstetric general anaesthesia: A literature review. International Journal of Obstetric Anesthesia. 2015;**24**(4):356-374

[9] Samsoon GL, Young JR. Difficult tracheal intubation: A retrospective study. Anaesthesia. 1987;**42**(5):487-490

[10] Palanisamy A, Mitani AA, Tsen LC. General anesthesia for cesarean delivery at a tertiary care hospital from 2000 to 2005: A retrospective analysis and 10-year update. International Journal of Obstetric Anesthesia. 2011;**20**(1):10-16

[11] Sealey JE, Itskovitz-Eldor J, Rubattu S, James GD, August P, Thaler I, et al. Estradiol-and progesterone-related increases in the renin-aldosterone system: Studies during ovarian stimulation and early pregnancy. The Journal of Clinical Endocrinology & Metabolism. 1994;**79**(1):258-264

[12] Lumbers ER, Pringle KG. Roles of the circulating renin-angiotensin-aldosterone system in human pregnancy. American Journal of Physiology-Regulatory, Integrative and Comparative Physiology. 2014;**306**(2):R91-R101

[13] Kodali BS, Chandrasekhar S, Bulich LN, Topulos GP, Datta S. Airway changes during labor and delivery. The Journal of the American Society of Anesthesiologists. 2008;**108**(3):357-362

[14] Boutonnet M, Faitot V, Katz A, Salomon L, Keita H. Mallampati class changes during pregnancy, labour, and after delivery: Can these be predicted? British Journal of Anaesthesia. 2010;**104**(1):67-70

[15] Jouppila R, Jouppila P, Hollmen A. Laryngeal oedema as an obstetric anaesthesia complication. Acta Anaesthesiologica Scandinavica. 1980;**24**(2):97-98

[16] Rocke DA, Murray WB, Rout CC, Gouws E. Relative risk analysis of factors associated with difficult intubation in obstetric anesthesia. The Journal of the American Society of Anesthesiologists. 1992;**77**(1):67-73

[17] Arendt KW, Khan K, Curry TB, Tsen LC. Topical vasoconstrictor use for nasal intubation during pregnancy complicated by cardiomyopathy and preeclampsia. International Journal of Obstetric Anesthesia. 2011;**20**(3):246-249

[18] Cunningham FG, Leveno KJ, Dashe JS, Hoffman BL, Spong CY, Casey BM. Williams Obstetrics. 26th ed. New York, NY, USA: Mcgraw-Hill; 2022

[19] Crapo RO. Normal cardiopulmonary physiology during pregnancy. Clinical Obstetrics and Gynecology. 1996;**39**(1):3-16

[20] Russell IF, Chambers WA. Closing volume in normal pregnancy. British Journal of Anaesthesia. 1981;**53**(10):1043-1047

[21] Weinberger SE, Weiss ST, Cohen WR, Weiss JW, Johnson TS. Pregnancy and the lung. American Review of Respiratory Disease. 1980;**121**(3):559-581

[22] Contreras G, GutiéRrez M, Beroíza T, Fantín A, Oddó H, Villarroel L, et al. Ventilatory drive and respiratory muscle function in pregnancy. American Review of Respiratory Disease. 2012;**144**(4):838-841

[23] McGinty AP. The comparative effects of pregnancy and phrenic nerve interruption on the diaphragm and their relation to pulmonary tuberculosis. American Journal of Obstetrics and Gynecology. 1938;**35**(2):237-248

[24] Gilroy RJ, Mangura BT, Lavietes MH. Rib cage and abdominal volume displacements during breathing in pregnancy. The American Review of Respiratory Disease. 1988;**137**:668-672

[25] Archer GW Jr, Marx GF. Arterial oxygen tension during apnoea in parturient women. British Journal of Anaesthesia. 1974;**46**(5):358-360

[26] Carstoniu J, Levytam S, Norman P, Daley D, Katz J, Sandler AN. Nitrous oxide in early labor safety and analgesic efficacy assessed by a double-blind, placebo-controlled study. Anesthesiology. 1994;**80**:30-35

[27] Wong CA, McCarthy RJ, Fitzgerald PC, Raikoff K, Avram MJ. Gastric emptying of water in obese pregnant women at term. Anesthesia & Analgesia. 2007;**105**(3):751-755

[28] Apfelbaum JL, Hagberg CA, Connis RT, Abdelmalak BB, Agarkar M, Dutton RP, et al. 2022 American Society of Anesthesiologists practice guidelines for management of the difficult airway. Anesthesiology. 2022;**136**(1):31-81

[29] Law JA, Duggan LV, Asselin M, Baker P, Crosby E, Downey A, et al. Canadian airway focus group updated consensus-based recommendations for management of the difficult airway: Part 1. Difficult airway management encountered in an unconscious patient. Canadian Journal of Anesthesia/ Journal canadien d'anesthésie. 2021;**68**(9):1373-1404

[30] Lundstrøm LH, Møller AM, Rosenstock C, Astrup G, Gätke MR, Wetterslev J, et al. A documented previous difficult tracheal intubation

as a prognostic test for a subsequent difficult tracheal intubation in adults. Anaesthesia. 2009;**64**(10):1081-1088

[31] Kheterpal S, Han R, Tremper KK, Shanks A, Tait AR, O'Reilly M, et al. Incidence and predictors of difficult and impossible mask ventilation. The Journal of the American Society of Anesthesiologists. 2006;**105**(5):885-891

[32] Yildiz TS, Solak M, Toker K. The incidence and risk factors of difficult mask ventilation. Journal of Anesthesia. 2005;**19**(1):7-11

[33] Gonzalez H, Minville V, Delanoue K, Mazerolles M, Concina D, Fourcade O. The importance of increased neck circumference to intubation difficulties in obese patients. Anesthesia & Analgesia. 2008;**106**(4):1132-1136

[34] Updated by the Committee on Standards and Practice Parameters, Apfelbaum JL, Hagberg CA, Caplan RA, Blitt CD, Connis RT, et al. Practice guidelines for management of the difficult airway: an updated report by the American Society of Anesthesiologists Task Force on Management of the Difficult Airway. Anesthesiology. 2013;**118**(2):251-270

[35] Shiga T, Wajima ZI, Inoue T, Sakamoto A. Predicting difficult intubation in apparently normal patients: A meta-analysis of bedside screening test performance. The Journal of the American Society of Anesthesiologists. 2005;**103**(2):429-437

[36] Mashour GA, Kheterpal S, Vanaharam V, Shanks A, Wang LY, Sandberg WS, et al. The extended Mallampati score and a diagnosis of diabetes mellitus are predictors of difficult laryngoscopy in the morbidly obese. Anesthesia & Analgesia. 2008;**107**(6):1919-1923

[37] Racine SX, Solis A, Hamou NA, Letoumelin P, Hepner DL, Beloucif S, et al. Face mask ventilation in edentulous patients: A comparison of mandibular groove and lower lip placement. The Journal of the American Society of Anesthesiologists. 2010;**112**(5):1190-1193

[38] Brodsky JB, Lemmens HJ, Brock-Utne JG, Vierra M, Saidman LJ. Morbid obesity and tracheal intubation. Anesthesia & Analgesia. 2002;**94**(3):732-736

[39] Lee A, Fan LT, Gin T, Karmakar MK, Kee WD. A systematic review (meta-analysis) of the accuracy of the Mallampati tests to predict the difficult airway. Anesthesia & Analgesia. 2006;**102**(6):1867-1878

[40] Lee A, Kee WD, Gin T. A quantitative, systematic review of randomized controlled trials of ephedrine versus phenylephrine for the management of hypotension during spinal anesthesia for cesarean delivery. Anesthesia & Analgesia. 2002;**94**(4):920-926

[41] Iohom G, Ronayne M, Cunningham AJ. Prediction of difficult tracheal intubation. European Journal of Anaesthesiology. 2003;**20**(1):31-36

[42] Wilson ME, Spiegelhalter D, Robertson JA, Lesser P. Predicting difficult intubation. British Journal of Anaesthesia. 1988;**61**(2):211-216

[43] Calder I, Calder J, Crockard HA. Difficult direct laryngoscopy in patients with cervical spine disease. Anaesthesia. 1995;**50**(9):756-763

[44] Khan ZH, Mohammadi M, Rasouli MR, Farrokhnia F, Khan RH. The diagnostic value of the upper lip bite test combined with sternomental

distance, thyromental distance, and interincisor distance for prediction of easy laryngoscopy and intubation: A prospective study. Anesthesia & Analgesia. 2009;**109**(3):822-824

[45] Khan ZH, Kashfi A, Ebrahimkhani E. A comparison of the upper lip bite test (a simple new technique) with modified Mallampati classification in predicting difficulty in endotracheal intubation: A prospective blinded study. Anesthesia & Analgesia. 2003;**96**(2):595-599

[46] Tygart SG, McRoyan DK, Spinnato JA, McRoyan CJ, Kitay DZ. Longitudinal study of platelet indices during normal pregnancy. American Journal of Obstetrics and Gynecology. 1986;**154**(4):883-887

[47] Ngan Kee WD, Khaw KS, Ng FF. Comparison of phenylephrine infusion regimens for maintaining maternal blood pressure during spinal anaesthesia for Caesarean section. British Journal of Anaesthesia. 2004;**92**(4):469-474

[48] Moslemi F, Khan ZH, Alizadeh E, Khamnian Z, Eftekhar N, Hosseini MS, et al. Upper lip bite test compared to modified Mallampati test in predicting difficult airway in obstetrics: A prospective observational study. Journal of Perioperative Practice. 2021:3-5

[49] Mushambi MC, Kinsella SM, Popat M, Swales H, Ramaswamy KK, Winton AL, et al. Obstetric Anaesthetists' Association and Difficult Airway Society guidelines for the management of difficult and failed tracheal intubation in obstetrics. Anaesthesia. 2015;**70**(11):1286-1306

[50] Frerk C, Mitchell VS, McNarry AF, Mendonca C, Bhagrath R, Patel A, et al. Difficult airway society 2015 guidelines for management of unanticipated difficult intubation in adults. British Journal of Anaesthesia. 2015;**115**(6):827-848

[51] Committee on Obstetric Practice. ACOG Committee Opinion No. 441. Oral intake during labor. Obstetrics & Gynecology. 2009;**114**(3):714

[52] Association of Anaesthetists of Great Britain and Ireland. Pre-Operative Assessment and Patient Preparation. The Role of the Anaesthetist 2. London: AAGBI; 2010

[53] National Collaborating Centre for Women's and Children's Health (UK). Intrapartum Care: Care of Healthy Women and Their Babies During Child Birth. NICE Clinical Guidelines. London: National Institute for Health and Care Excellence; 2014

[54] Practice Guidelines for Preoperative Fasting and the Use of Pharmacologic Agents to Reduce the Risk of Pulmonary Aspiration. Application to healthy patients undergoing elective procedures: An updated report by the American Society of Anesthesiologists Task Force on preoperative fasting and the use of pharmacologic agents to reduce the risk of pulmonary aspiration. Anesthesiology. 2017;**126**(3):376-393

[55] Artime CA, Sanchez A. Preparation of the patient for awake intubation. In: Hagberg and Benumof's Airway Management. 4th ed. Philadelphia, PA: Elsevier; 2018. pp. p216-p234

[56] Schneck H, Scheller M. Acid aspiration prophylaxis and caesarean section. Current Opinion in Anesthesiology. 2000;**13**(3):261-265

[57] Paranjothy S, Griffiths JD, Broughton HK, et al. Interventions at caesarean section for reducing the risk of aspiration pneumonitis. Cochrane Database of Systematic Reviews. 2010;**2020**(1):CD004943

[58] Paranjothy S, Griffiths JD, Broughton HK, Gyte GM, Brown HC, Thomas J. Interventions at caesarean section for reducing the risk of aspiration pneumonitis. International Journal of Obstetric Anesthesia. 2011;**20**(2):142-148

[59] O'Sullican GM, Bullingham RE. The assessment of gastric acidity and antacid effect in pregnant women by a non-invasive radiotelemetry technique. BJOG: An International Journal of Obstetrics & Gynaecology. 1984;**91**(10):973-978

[60] El-Orbany M, Connolly LA. Rapid sequence induction and intubation: Current controversy. Anesthesia & Analgesia. 2010;**110**(5):1318-1325

[61] Koerber JP, Roberts GE, Whitaker R, Thorpe CM. Variation in rapid sequence induction techniques: Current practice in Wales. Anaesthesia. 2009;**64**(1):54-59

[62] Rosen MA, Weiskopf RB. Management of anesthesia for the pregnant surgical patient. The Journal of the American Society of Anesthesiologists. 1999;**91**(4):1159

[63] Brown JP, Werrett GC. Bag-mask ventilation in rapid sequence induction: A survey of current practice among members of the UK difficult airway society. European Journal of Anaesthesiology| EJA. 2015;**32**(6):446-448

[64] Gal TJ. Airway management. In: Miller RD, editor. Miller's Anesthesia. 6th ed. Philadelphia: Churchill Livingstone; 2005. pp. 1617-1652

[65] Donati F. The right dose of succinylcholine. The Journal of the American Society of Anesthesiologists. 2003;**99**(5):1037-1038

[66] Naguib M, Samarkandi AH, El-Din ME, Abdullah K, Khaled M, Alharby SW. The dose of succinylcholine required for excellent endotracheal intubating conditions. Anesthesia & Analgesia. 2006;**102**(1):151-155

[67] Naguib M, Samarkandi A, Riad W, Alharby SW. Optimal dose of succinylcholine revisited. The Journal of the American Society of Anesthesiologists. 2003;**99**(5):1045-1049

[68] Blitt CD, Petty WC, Alberternst EE, Wright BJ. Correlation of plasma cholinesterase activity and duration of action of succinylcholine during pregnancy. Anesthesia and Analgesia. 1977;**56**(1):78-83

[69] Deepika K, Bikhazi GB, Mikati HM, Namba M, Foldes FF. Facilitation of rapid-sequence intuhation with large-dose vecuronium with or without priming. Journal of Clinical Anesthesia. 1992;**4**(2):106-110

[70] Williamson RM, Mallaiah S, Barclay P. Rocuronium and sugammadex for rapid sequence induction of obstetric general anaesthesia. Acta Anaesthesiologica Scandinavica. 2011;**55**(6):694-699

[71] Abu-Halaweh SA, Massad IM, Abu-Ali HM, Badran IZ, Barazangi BA, Ramsay MA. Rapid sequence induction and intubation with 1 mg/kg rocuronium bromide in cesarean section, comparison with suxamethonium. Saudi Medical Journal. 2007;**28**(9):1393-1396

[72] Sørensen MK, Bretlau C, Gätke MR, Sørensen AM, Rasmussen LS. Rapid sequence induction and intubation with rocuronium–sugammadex compared with succinylcholine: A randomized trial. British Journal of Anaesthesia. 2012;**108**(4):682-689

[73] Fuchs-Buder T, Schmartz D. The never ending story or the search for a nondepolarising alternative to

succinylcholine. European Journal of Anaesthesiology. 2013;**30**(10):583-584

[74] Girard T. Pro: Rocuronium should replace succinylcholine for rapid sequence induction. European Journal of Anaesthesiology. 2013;**30**(10):585-589

[75] Naguib M. Sugammadex: Another milestone in clinical neuromuscular pharmacology. Anesthesia & Analgesia. 2007;**104**(3):575-581

[76] Naguib M, Kopman AF, Lien CA, Hunter JM, Lopez A, Brull SJ. A survey of current management of neuromuscular block in the United States and Europe. Anesthesia & Analgesia. 2010;**111**(1):110-119

[77] Lawes EG, Campbell I, Mercer D. Inflation pressure, gastric insufflation and rapid sequence induction. British Journal of Anaesthesia. 1987;**59**(3):315-318

[78] Petito SP, Russell WJ. The prevention of gastric inflation—A neglected benefit of cricoid pressure. Anaesthesia and Intensive Care. 1988;**16**(2):139-143

[79] Swales H, Mushambi M, Winton A, Ramaswamy K, Quinn A, Kinsella M. Management of failed intubation and difficult airways in UK obstetric units: An OAA survey. International Journal of Obstetric Anesthesia. 2014;**23** (Suppl. 1):S19

[80] Zaouter C, Calderon J, Hemmerling TM. Videolaryngoscopy as a new standard of care. British Journal of Anaesthesia. 2015;**114**(2):181-183

[81] Dhonneur G, Ndoko S, Amathieu R, Housseini LE, Poncelet C, Tual L. Tracheal intubation using the Airtraq® in morbid obese patients undergoing emergency cesarean delivery. The Journal of the American Society of Anesthesiologists. 2007;**106**(3):629-630

[82] Riad W, Ansari T. Effect of cricoid pressure on the laryngoscopic view by Airtraq in elective caesarean section: A pilot study. European Journal of Anaesthesiology. 2009;**26**(11):981-982

[83] Turkstra TP, Armstrong PM, Jones PM, Quach T. GlideScope® use in the obstetric patient. International Journal of Obstetric Anesthesia. 2010;**19**(1):123-124

[84] Shonfeld A, Gray K, Lucas N, Robinson N, Loughnan B, Morris H, et al. Video laryngoscopy in obstetric anesthesia. Journal of Obstetric Anaesthesia and Critical Care. 2012;**2**(1):53

[85] Arici S, Karaman S, Doğru S, Karaman T, Tapar H, Özsoy AZ, et al. The McGrath series 5 video laryngoscope versus the Macintosh laryngoscope: A randomized trial in obstetric patients. Turkish Journal of Medical Sciences. 2014;**44**(3):387-392

[86] Aziz MF, Kim D, Mako J, Hand K, Brambrink AM. A retrospective study of the performance of video laryngoscopy in an obstetric unit. Anesthesia & Analgesia. 2012;**115**(4):904-906

[87] Mustapha B, Chkoura K, Elhassani M, Ahtil R, Azendour H, Kamili ND. Difficult intubation in a parturient with syringomyelia and Arnold–Chiari malformation: Use of Airtraq™ laryngoscope. Saudi Journal of Anaesthesia. 2011;**5**(4):419

[88] Ni J, Luo L, Wu L, Luo D. The Airtraq™ laryngoscope as a first choice for parturients with an expected difficult airway. International Journal of Obstetric Anesthesia. 2014;**23**(1):94-95

[89] Browning RM, Rucklidge MW. Tracheal intubation using the Pentax

airway scope videolaryngoscope following failed direct laryngoscopy in a morbidly obese parturient. International Journal of Obstetric Anesthesia. 2011;**20**(2):200-201

[90] Tonidandel A, Booth J, D'angelo R, Harris L, Tonidandel S. Anesthetic and obstetric outcomes in morbidly obese parturients: A 20-year follow-up retrospective cohort study. International Journal of Obstetric Anesthesia. 2014;**23**(4):357-364

[91] Benumof JL, Cooper SD. Quantitative improvement in laryngoscopic view by optimal external laryngeal manipulation. Journal of Clinical Anesthesia. 1996;**8**(2):136-140

[92] Latto IP, Stacey M, Mecklenburgh J, Vaughan RS. Survey of the use of the gum elastic bougie in clinical practice. Anaesthesia. 2002;**57**(4):379-384

[93] Hodzovic I, Latto IP, Henderson JJ. Bougie trauma--What trauma? Anaesthesia. 2003;**58**(2):192-193

[94] Kadry M, Popat M. Pharyngeal wall perforation—An unusual complication of blind intubation with a gum elastic bougic. Anaesthesia. 1999;**54**(4):404-405

[95] Arndt GA, Cambray AJ, Tomasson J. Intubation bougie dissection of tracheal mucosa and intratracheal airway obstruction. Anesthesia & Analgesia. 2008;**107**(2):603-604

[96] Pandit JJ, Andrade J, Bogod DG, Hitchman JM, Jonker WR, Lucas N, et al. 5th National Audit Project (NAP5) on accidental awareness during general anaesthesia: Summary of main findings and risk factors. British journal of anaesthesia. 2014;**69**:1089-1101

[97] Odor PM, Bampoe S, Moonesinghe SR, Andrade J, Pandit JJ, Lucas DN. Pan-London perioperative audit and research network (PLAN), for the DREAMY investigators group, A'Court A, Abdel-Gadir D, Abdu A, Abisogun C. General anaesthetic and airway management practice for obstetric surgery in England: A prospective, multicentre observational study. Anaesthesia. 2021;**76**(4):460-471

[98] Sakles JC, Patanwala AE, Mosier JM, Dicken JM. Comparison of video laryngoscopy to direct laryngoscopy for intubation of patients with difficult airway characteristics in the emergency department. Internal and Emergency Medicine. 2014;**9**(1):93-98

[99] Mosier JM, Stolz U, Chiu S, Sakles JC. Difficult airway management in the emergency department: GlideScope videolaryngoscopy compared to direct laryngoscopy. The Journal of Emergency Medicine. 2012;**42**(6):629-634

[100] Park R, Peyton JM, Fiadjoe JE, Hunyady AI, Kimball T, Zurakowski D, et al. TheefficacyofGlideScope® videolaryngoscopy compared with direct laryngoscopy in children who are difficult to intubate: An analysis from the paediatric difficult intubation registry. BJA: British Journal of Anaesthesia. 2017;**119**(5):984-992

[101] Dillon JK, Christensen B, Fairbanks T, Jurkovich G, Moe KS. The emergent surgical airway: Cricothyrotomy vs tracheotomy. International Journal of Oral and Maxillofacial Surgery. 2013;**42**(2):204-208

[102] Kristensen MS, Teoh WH, Baker PA. Percutaneous emergency airway access; prevention, preparation, technique and training. British Journal of Anaesthesia. 2015;**114**(3):357-361

[103] Royal College of Obstetricians & Gynaecologists. Maternal collapse in pregnancy and the puerperium. Green Top Guideline. 2011;(56):2-6

[104] Law JA, Duggan LV, Asselin M, Baker P, Crosby E, Downey A, et al. Canadian airway focus group updated consensus-based recommendations for management of the difficult airway: Part 2. Planning and implementing safe management of the patient with an anticipated difficult airway. Canadian Journal of Anesthesia/Journal canadien d'anesthésie. 2021;**68**(9):1405-1436

[105] McDonnell NJ, Paech MJ, Clavisi OM, Scott KL, ANZCA Trials Group. Difficult and failed intubation in obstetric anaesthesia: An observational study of airway management and complications associated with general anaesthesia for caesarean section. International journal of obstetric anesthesia. 2008;**17**(4):292-297

[106] Malik D, Mushambi M, Ali P, Dravid MR. Tracheal extubation practices amongst members of the difficult airway society: A national survey. Anaesthesia. 2013;**68**(6):656-656 111 River St, Hoboken 07030-5774, NJ, USA: Wiley-Blackwell